Hard Press

THE ANALECTS OF CONFUCIUS

Introduction

BOOK

THE SAYINGS OF MENCIUS

THE SHI-KING

THE SORROWS OF HAN

THE ANALECTS

OF

CONFUCIUS

[*Translated into English by William Jennings*]

PRONUNCIATION OF PROPER NAMES

j, as in French. *ng*, commencing a word, like the same letters terminating one. *ai* or *ei*, as in *aisle* or *eider*. *au*, as in German, or like *ow* in *cow*. *e*, as in *fête*. *i* (not followed by a consonant), as *ee* in *see*. *u* (followed by a consonant), as in *bull*. *iu*, as *ew* in *new*. *ui*, as *ooi* in *cooing*. *h* at the end of a name makes the preceding vowel short. *i* in the middle of a word denotes an aspirate (*h*), as *K'ung*=Khung.

INTRODUCTION

The strangest figure that meets us in the annals of Oriental thought is that of Confucius. To the popular mind he is the founder of a religion, and yet he has nothing in common with the great religious teachers of the East. We think of Siddartha, the founder of Buddhism, as the very impersonation of romantic asceticism, enthusiastic self-sacrifice, and faith in the things that are invisible. Zoroaster is the friend of God, talking face to face with the Almighty, and drinking wisdom and knowledge from the lips of Omniscience. Mohammed is represented as snatched up into heaven, where he receives the Divine communication which he is bidden to propagate with fire and sword throughout the world. These great teachers lived in an atmosphere of the supernatural. They spoke with the authority of inspired prophets. They brought the unseen world close to the minds of their disciples. They spoke positively of immortality, of reward or punishment beyond the grave. The present life they despised, the future was to them everything in its promised satisfaction. The teachings of Confucius were of a very different sort. Throughout his whole writings he has not even mentioned the name of God. He declined to discuss the question of immortality. When he was asked about spiritual beings, he remarked, "If we cannot even know men, how can we know spirits?"

Yet this was the man the impress of whose teaching has formed the national character of five hundred millions of people. A temple to Confucius stands to this day in every town and village of China. His precepts are committed to memory by every child from the tenderest age, and each year at the royal university at Pekin the Emperor holds a festival in honor of the illustrious teacher.

The influence of Confucius springs, first of all, from the narrowness and definiteness of his doctrine. He was no transcendentalist, and never meddled with supramundane things. His teaching was of the earth, earthy; it dealt entirely with the common relations of life, and the Golden Rule he must necessarily have stumbled upon, as the most obvious canon of his system. He strikes us as being the great Stoic of the East, for he believed that virtue was based on knowledge, knowledge of a man's own heart, and knowledge of human-kind. There is a pathetic resemblance between the accounts given of the death of Confucius and the death of Zeno. Both died almost without warning in dreary hopelessness, without the ministrations of either love or religion. This may be a mere coincidence, but the lives and teachings of both men must have led them to look with indifference upon such an end. For Confucius in his teaching treated only of man's life on earth, and seems to have had no ideas with regard to the human lot after death; if he had any ideas he preserved an inscrutable silence about them. As a moralist he prescribed the duties of the king and of the father, and advocated the cultivation by the individual man of that rest or apathy of mind which resembles so much the disposition aimed at by the Greek and Roman Stoic. Even as a moralist, he seems to have sacrificed the ideal to the practical, and his loose notions about marriage, his tolerance of concubinage, the slight emphasis which he lays on the virtue of veracity—of which indeed he does not seem himself to have been particularly studious in his historic writings—place him low down in the rank of moralists. Yet he taught what he felt the people could receive, and the flat mediocrity of his character and his teachings has been stamped forever upon a people who, while they are kindly, gentle, forbearing, and full of family piety, are palpably lacking not only in the exaltation of Mysticism, but in any religious feeling, generally so-called.

The second reason that made the teaching of Confucius so influential is based on the circumstances of the time. When this thoughtful, earnest youth awoke to the consciousness of life about him, he saw that the abuses under which the people groaned sprang from the feudal system, which cut up the country into separate territories, over which the power of the king had no control. China was in the position of France in the years preceding Philippe-Auguste, excepting that there were no places of sanctuary and no Truce of God. The great doctrine of Confucius was the unlimited despotism of the Emperor, and his moral precepts were intended to teach the Emperor how to use his power aright. But the Emperor was only typical of all those in authority—the feudal duke, the judge on the bench, and the father of the family. Each could discharge his duties aright only by submitting to the moral discipline which Confucius prescribed. A vital element in this system is its conservatism, its adherence to the imperial idea. As James I said, "No bishop, no king," so the imperialists of China have found in Confucianism the strongest basis for the throne, and have supported its dissemination accordingly.

The Analects of Confucius contain the gist of his teachings, and is worthy of study. We find in this work most of the precepts which his disciples have preserved and recorded. They form a code remarkable for simplicity, even crudity, and we are compelled to admire the force of character, the practical sagacity, the insight into the needs of the hour, which enabled Confucius, without claiming any Divine sanction, to impose this system upon his countrymen.

The name Confucius is only the Latinized form of two words which mean "Master K'ung." He was born 551 B.C., his father being governor of Shantung. He was married at nineteen, and seems to have occupied some minor position under the government. In his twenty-fourth year he entered upon the three years' mourning for the death of his mother. His seclusion gave him time for deep thought and the study of history, and he resolved upon the regeneration of his unhappy country. By the time he was thirty he became known as a great teacher, and disciples flocked to him. But he was yet occupied in public duties, and rose through successive stages to the office of Chief Judge in his own country of Lu. His tenure of office is said to have put an end to crime, and he became the "idol of the people" in his district. The jealousy of the feudal lords was roused by his fame as a moral teacher and a blameless judge. Confucius was driven from his home, and wandered about, with a few disciples, until his sixty-ninth year, when he returned to Lu, after accomplishing a work which has borne fruit, such as it is, to the present day. He spent the remaining five years of his life in editing the odes and historic monuments in which the glories of the ancient Chinese dynasty are set forth. He died in his seventy-third year, 478 B.C. There can be no doubt that the success of Confucius has been singularly great, owing especially to the narrow scope of his scheme, which has become crystallized in the habits, usages, and customs of the people. Especially has it been instrumental in consolidating the empire, and in strengthening the power of the monarch, who, as he every year burns incense in the red-walled temple at Pekin, utters sincerely the invocation: "Great art thou, O perfect Sage! Thy virtue is full, thy doctrine complete. Among mortal men there has not been thine equal. All kings honor thee. Thy statutes and laws have come gloriously down. Thou art the pattern in this imperial school. Reverently have the sacrificial vessels been set out. Full of awe, we sound our drums and bells."

E. W.

BOOK I

On Learning—Miscellaneous Sayings:—

"To learn," said the Master, "and then to practise opportunely what one has learnt—does not this bring with it a sense of satisfaction?

"To have associates in study coming to one from distant parts—does not this also mean pleasure in store?

"And are not those who, while not comprehending all that is said, still remain not unpleased to hear, men of the superior order?"

A saying of the Scholar Yu:—

"It is rarely the case that those who act the part of true men in regard to their duty to parents and elder brothers are at the same time willing to turn currishly upon their superiors: it has never yet been the case that such as desire not to commit that offence have been men willing to promote anarchy or disorder.

"Men of superior mind busy themselves first in getting at the root of things; and when they have succeeded in this the right course is open to them. Well, are not filial piety and friendly subordination among brothers a root of that right feeling which is owing generally from man to man?"

The Master observed, "Rarely do we meet with the right feeling due from one man to another where there is fine speech and studied mien."

The Scholar Tsang once said of himself: "On three points I examine myself daily, *viz.*, whether, in looking after other people's interests, I have not been acting whole-heartedly; whether, in my intercourse with friends, I have not been true; and whether, after teaching, I have not myself been practising what I have taught."

The Master once observed that to rule well one of the larger States meant strict attention to its affairs and conscientiousness on the part of the ruler; careful husbanding of its resources, with at the same time a tender care for the interests of all classes; and the employing of the masses in the public service at suitable seasons.

"Let young people," said he, "show filial piety at home, respectfulness towards their elders when away from home; let them be circumspect, be truthful; their love going out freely towards all, cultivating good-will to men. And if, in such a walk, there be time or energy left for other things, let them employ it in the acquisition of literary or artistic accomplishments."

The disciple Tsz-hia said, "The appreciation of worth in men of worth, thus diverting the mind from lascivious desires—ministering to parents while one is the most capable of so doing—serving one's ruler when one is able to devote himself entirely to that object—being sincere in one's language in intercourse with friends: this I certainly must call evidence of learning, though others may say there has been 'no learning.'"

Sayings of the Master:—

"If the great man be not grave, he will not be revered, neither can his learning be solid.

"Give prominent place to loyalty and sincerity.

"Have no associates in study who are not advanced somewhat like yourself.

"When you have erred, be not afraid to correct yourself."

A saying of the Scholar Tsang:—

"The virtue of the people is renewed and enriched when attention is seen to be paid to the departed, and the remembrance of distant ancestors kept and cherished."

Tsz-k'in put this query to his fellow disciple Tsz-kung: said he, "When our Master comes to this or that State, he learns without fail how it is being governed. Does he investigate matters? or are the facts given him?"

Tsz-kung answered, "Our Master is a man of pleasant manners, and of probity, courteous, moderate, and unassuming: it is by his being such that he arrives at the facts. Is not his way of arriving at things different from that of others?"

A saying of the Master:—

"He who, after three years' observation of the will of his father when alive, or of his past conduct if dead, does not deviate from that father's ways, is entitled to be called 'a dutiful son.'"

Sayings of the Scholar Yu:—

"For the practice of the Rules of Propriety,[1] one excellent way is to be natural. This naturalness became a great grace in the practice of kings of former times; let everyone, small or great, follow their example.

"It is not, however, always practicable; and it is not so in the case of a person who does things naturally, knowing that he should act so, and yet who neglects to regulate his acts according to the Rules.

"When truth and right are hand in hand, a statement will bear repetition. When respectfulness and propriety go hand in hand, disgrace and shame are kept afar-off. Remove all occasion for alienating those to whom you are bound by close ties, and you have them still to resort to."

A saying of the Master:—

"The man of greater mind who, when he is eating, craves not to eat to the full; who has a home, but craves not for comforts in it; who is active and earnest in his work and careful in his words; who makes towards men of high principle, and so maintains his own rectitude—that man may be styled a devoted student."

Tsz-kung asked, "What say you, sir, of the poor who do not cringe and fawn; and what of the rich who are without pride and haughtiness?" "They are passable," the Master replied; "yet they are scarcely in the same category as the poor who are happy, and the rich who love propriety."

"In the 'Book of the Odes,'" Tsz-kung went on to say, "we read of one

Polished, as by the knife and file,
The graving-tool, the smoothing-stone.

Does that coincide with your remark?"

"Ah! such as you," replied the Master, "may well commence a discussion on the Odes. If one tell you how a thing goes, you know what ought to come."

"It does not greatly concern me," said the Master, "that men do not know me; my great concern is, my not knowing them."

[Footnote 1: An important part of a Chinaman's education still. The text-book, "The Li Ki," contains rules for behavior and propriety for the whole life, from the cradle to the grave.]

BOOK II

Good Government—Filial Piety—The Superior Man

Sayings of the Master:—

"Let a ruler base his government upon virtuous principles, and he will be like the pole-star, which remains steadfast in its place, while all the host of stars turn towards it.

"The 'Book of Odes' contains three hundred pieces, but one expression in it may be taken as covering the purport of all, *viz.*, Unswerving mindfulness.

"To govern simply by statute, and to reduce all to order by means of pains and penalties, is to render the people evasive, and devoid of any sense of shame.

"To govern upon principles of virtue, and to reduce them to order by the Rules of Propriety, would not only create in them the sense of shame, but would moreover reach them in all their errors.

"When I attained the age of fifteen, I became bent upon study. At thirty, I was a confirmed student. At forty, nought could move me from my course. At fifty, I comprehended the will and decrees of Heaven. At sixty, my ears were attuned to them. At seventy, I could follow my heart's desires, without overstepping the lines of rectitude."

To a question of Mang-i, as to what filial piety consisted in, the master replied, "In not being perverse." Afterwards, when Fan Ch'i was driving him, the Master informed him of this question and answer, and Fan Ch'i asked, "What was your meaning?" The Master replied, "I meant that the Rules of Propriety should always be adhered to in regard to those who brought us into the world: in ministering to them while living, in burying them when dead, and afterwards in the offering to them of sacrificial gifts."

To a query of Mang Wu respecting filial piety, the Master replied, "Parents ought to bear but one trouble—that of their own sickness."

To a like question put by Tsz-yu, his reply was this: "The filial piety of the present day simply means the being able to support one's parents—which extends even to the case of dogs and horses, all of which may have something to give in the way of support. If there be no reverential feeling in the matter, what is there to distinguish between the cases?"

To a like question of Tsz-hia, he replied: "The manner is the difficulty. If, in the case of work to be done, the younger folks simply take upon themselves the toil of it;

or if, in the matter of meat and drink, they simply set these before their elders—is this to be taken as filial piety?"

Once the Master remarked, "I have conversed with Hwui the whole day long, and he has controverted nothing that I have said, as if he were without wits. But when his back was turned, and I looked attentively at his conduct apart from me, I found it satisfactory in all its issues. No, indeed! Hwui is not without his wits."

Other observations of the Master:—

"If you observe what things people (usually) take in hand, watch their motives, and note particularly what it is that gives them satisfaction, shall they be able to conceal from you what they are? Conceal themselves, indeed!

"Be versed in ancient lore, and familiarize yourself with the modern; then may you become teachers.

"The great man is not a mere receptacle."

In reply to Tsz-kung respecting the great man:—

"What he first says, as a result of his experience, he afterwards follows up.

"The great man is catholic-minded, and not one-sided. The common man is the reverse.

"Learning, without thought, is a snare; thought, without learning, is a danger.

"Where the mind is set much upon heterodox principles—there truly and indeed is harm."

To the disciple Tsz-lu the Master said, "Shall I give you a lesson about knowledge? When you know a thing, maintain that you know it; and when you do not, acknowledge your ignorance. This is characteristic of knowledge."

Tsz-chang was studying with an eye to official income. The Master addressed him thus: "Of the many things you hear hold aloof from those that are doubtful, and speak guardedly with reference to the rest; your mistakes will then be few. Also, of the many courses you see adopted, hold aloof from those that are risky, and carefully follow the others; you will then seldom have occasion for regret. Thus, being seldom mistaken in your utterances, and having few occasions for regret in the line you take, you are on the high road to your preferment."

To a question put to him by Duke Ngai [2] as to what should be done in order to render the people submissive to authority, Confucius replied, "Promote the straightforward, and reject those whose courses are crooked, and the thing will be effected. Promote the crooked and reject the straightforward, and the effect will be the reverse."

When Ki K'ang [3] asked of him how the people could be induced to show respect, loyalty, and willingness to be led, the Master answered, "Let there be grave dignity in him who has the oversight of them, and they will show him respect; let him be seen to be good to his own parents, and kindly in disposition, and they will be loyal to him; let him promote those who have ability, and see to the instruction of those who have it not, and they will be willing to be led."

Some one, speaking to Confucius, inquired, "Why, sir, are you not an administrator of government?" The Master rejoined, "What says the 'Book of the Annals,' with reference to filial duty?—'Make it a point to be dutiful to your parents and amicable with your brethren; the same duties extend to an administrator.' If these, then, also make an administrator, how am I to take your words about being an administrator?"

On one occasion the Master remarked, "I know not what men are good for, on whose word no reliance can be placed. How should your carriages, large or little, get along without your whipple-trees or swing-trees?"

Tsz-chang asked if it were possible to forecast the state of the country ten generations hence. The Master replied in this manner: "The Yin dynasty adopted the rules and manners of the Hia line of kings, and it is possible to tell whether it retrograded or advanced. The Chow line has followed the Yin, adopting its ways, and whether there has been deterioration or improvement may also be determined. Some other line may take up in turn those of Chow; and supposing even this process to go on for a hundred generations, the result may be known."

Other sayings of the Master:—

"It is but flattery to make sacrificial offerings to departed spirits not belonging to one's own family.

"It is moral cowardice to leave undone what one perceives to be right to do."

[Footnote 2: Of Lu (Confucius's native State).]

[Footnote 3: Head of one of the "Three Families" of Lu.]

BOOK III

Abuse of Proprieties in Ceremonial and Music

Alluding to the head of the Ki family, [4] and the eight lines of posturers [5] before their ancestral hall, Confucius remarked, "If the Ki can allow himself to go to this extent, to what extent will he not allow himself to go?"

The Three Families [6] were in the habit, during the Removal of the sacred vessels after sacrifice, of using the hymn commencing,

"Harmoniously the Princes
  Draw near with reverent tread,
Assisting in his worship
  Heaven's Son, the great and dread."

"How," exclaimed the Master, "can such words be appropriated in the ancestral hall of the Three Families?"

"Where a man," said he again, "has not the proper feelings due from one man to another, how will he stand as regards the Rules of Propriety? And in such a case, what shall we say of his sense of harmony?"

On a question being put to him by Lin Fang, a disciple, as to what was the radical idea upon which the Rules of Propriety were based, the Master exclaimed, "Ah! that is a large question. As to some rules, where there is likelihood of extravagance, they would rather demand economy; in those which relate to mourning, and where there is likelihood of being easily satisfied, what is wanted is real sorrow."

Speaking of the disorder of the times he remarked that while the barbarians on the North and East had their Chieftains, we here in this great country had nothing to compare with them in that respect:—we had lost these distinctions!

Alluding to the matter of the Chief of the Ki family worshipping on Tai-shan, [7] the Master said to Yen Yu, "Cannot you save him from this?" He replied, "It is beyond my power." "Alas, alas!" exclaimed the Master, "are we to say that the spirits of T'ai-shan have not as much discernment as Lin Fang?"

Of "the superior man," the Master observed, "In him there is no contentiousness. Say even that he does certainly contend with others, as in archery competitions; yet mark, in that case, how courteously he will bow and go up for the forfeit-cup, and come down again and give it to his competitor. In his very contest he is still the superior man."

Tsz-hia once inquired what inference might be drawn from the lines—

"Dimples playing in witching smile,
Beautiful eyes, so dark, so bright!
Oh, and her face may be thought the while
Colored by art, red rose on white!"

"Coloring," replied the Master, "requires a pure and clear background." "Then," said the other, "rules of ceremony require to have a background!" "Ah!" exclaimed the Master, "you are the man to catch the drift of my thought. Such as you may well introduce a discussion on the Odes."

Said the Master, "As regards the ceremonial adopted and enforced by the Hia dynasty, I am able to describe it, although their own descendants in the State of Ki can adduce no adequate testimony in favor of its use there. So, too, I am able to describe the ceremonial of the Yin dynasty, although no more can the Sung people show sufficient reason for its continuance amongst themselves. And why cannot they do so? Because they have not documents enough, nor men learned enough. If only they had such, I could refer them to them in support of their usages.

"When I am present at the great quinquennial sacrifice to the *manes* of the royal ancestors," the Master said, "from the pouring-out of the oblation onwards, I have no heart to look on."

Some one asked what was the purport of this great sacrifice, and the Master replied, "I cannot tell. The position in the empire of him who could tell you is as evident as when you look at this"—pointing to the palm of his hand.

When he offered sacrifices to his ancestors, he used to act as if they were present before him. In offering to other spirits it was the same.

He would say, "If I do not myself take part in my offerings, it is all the same as if I did not offer them."

Wang-sun Kia asked him once, "What says the proverb, 'Better to court favor in the kitchen than in the drawing-room'?" The Master replied, "Nay, better say, He who has sinned against Heaven has none other to whom prayer may be addressed."

Of the Chow dynasty the Master remarked, "It looks back upon two other dynasties; and what a rich possession it has in its records of those times! I follow Chow!"

On his first entry into the grand temple, he inquired about every matter connected with its usages. Some one thereupon remarked, "Who says that the son of the man of Tsou [8] understands about ceremonial? On entering the grand temple he inquired about everything." This remark coming to the Master's ears, he said, "What I did is part of the ceremonial!"

"In archery," he said, "the great point to be observed is not simply the perforation of the leather; for men have not all the same strength. That was the fashion in the olden days."

Once, seeing that his disciple Tsz-kung was desirous that the ceremonial observance of offering a sheep at the new moon might be dispensed with, the Master said, "Ah! you grudge the loss of the sheep; I grudge the loss of the ceremony."

"To serve one's ruler nowadays," he remarked, "fully complying with the Rules of Propriety, is regarded by others as toadyism!"

When Duke Ting questioned him as to how a prince should deal with his ministers, and how they in turn should serve their prince, Confucius said in reply, "In dealing with his ministers a prince should observe the proprieties; in serving his prince a minister should observe the duty of loyalty."

Referring to the First of the Odes, he remarked that it was mirthful without being lewd, and sad also without being painful.

Duke Ngai asked the disciple Tsai Wo respecting the places for sacrificing to the Earth. The latter replied, "The Family of the Great Yu, of the Hia dynasty, chose a place of pine trees; the Yin founders chose cypresses; and the Chow founders chestnut trees, solemn and majestic, to inspire, 'tis said, the people with feelings of awe."

The Master on hearing of this exclaimed, "Never an allusion to things that have been enacted in the past! Never a remonstrance against what is now going on! He has gone away without a word of censure."

The Master once said of Kwan Chung, [9] "A small-minded man indeed!"

"Was he miserly?" some one asked.

"Miserly, indeed!" said he; "not that: he married three rimes, and he was not a man who restricted his official business to too few hands—how could he be miserly?"

"He knew the Rules of Propriety, I suppose?"

"Judge:—Seeing that the feudal lords planted a screen at their gates, he too would have one at his! Seeing that when any two of the feudal lords met in friendly conclave they had an earthenware stand on which to place their inverted cups after drinking, he must have the same! If he knew the Rules of Propriety, who is there that does not know them?"

In a discourse to the Chief Preceptor of Music at the court of Lu, the Master said, "Music is an intelligible thing. When you begin a performance, let all the various instruments produce as it were one sound (inharmonious); then, as you go on, bring out the harmony fully, distinctly, and with uninterrupted flow, unto the end."

The warden of the border-town of I requested an interview with Confucius, and said, "When great men have come here, I have never yet failed to obtain a sight of them." The followers introduced him; and, on leaving, he said to them, "Sirs, why grieve at his loss of office? The empire has for long been without good government; and Heaven is about to use your master as its edict-announcer."

Comparing the music of the emperor Shun with the music of King Wu, the Master said, "That of Shun is beautiful throughout, and also good throughout. That of Wu is all of it beautiful, but scarcely all of it good."

"High station," said the Master, "occupied by men who have no large and generous heart; ceremonial performed with no reverence; duties of mourning engaging the attention, where there is absence of sorrow;—how should I look on, where this is the state of things?"

[Footnote 4: The Chief of the Ki clan was virtually the Duke of Lu, under whom Confucius for a time held office.]

[Footnote 5: These posturers were mutes who took part in the ritual of the ancestral temple, waving plumes, flags, *etc.* Each line or rank of these contained eight men. Only in the sovereign's household should there have been eight lines of them; a ducal family like the Ki should have had but six lines; a great official had four, and one of lower grade two. These were the gradations marking the status of families, and Confucius's sense of propriety was offended at the Ki's usurping in this way the appearance of royalty.]

[Footnote 6: Three great families related to each other, in whose hands the government of the State of Lu then was, and of which the Ki was the chief.]

[Footnote 7: One of the five sacred mountains, worshipped upon only by the sovereign.]

[Footnote 8: Tsou was Confucius's birthplace; his father was governor of the town.]

[Footnote 9: A renowned statesman who flourished about two hundred years before Confucius's time. A philosophical work on law and government, said to have been written by him, is still extant. He was regarded as a sage by the people, but he lacked, in Confucius's eyes, the one thing needful—propriety.]

BOOK IV

Social Virtue—Superior and Inferior Man

Sayings of the Master:—

"It is social good feeling that gives charm to a neighborhood. And where is the wisdom of those who choose an abode where it does not abide?

"Those who are without it cannot abide long, either in straitened or in happy circumstances. Those who possess it find contentment in it. Those who are wise go after it as men go after gain.

"Only they in whom it exists can have right likings and dislikings for others.

"Where the will is set upon it, there will be no room for malpractices.

"Riches and honor are what men desire; but if they arrive at them by improper ways, they should not continue to hold them. Poverty and low estate are what men dislike; but if they arrive at such a condition by improper ways, they should not refuse it.

"If the 'superior man' make nought of social good feeling, how shall he fully bear that name?

"Not even whilst he eats his meal will the 'superior man' forget what he owes to his fellow-men. Even in hurried leave-takings, even in moments of frantic confusion, he keeps true to this virtue.

"I have not yet seen a lover of philanthropy, nor a hater of misanthropy—such, that the former did not take occasion to magnify that virtue in himself, and that the latter, in his positive practice of philanthropy, did not, at times, allow in his presence something savoring of misanthropy.

"Say you, is there any one who is able for one whole day to apply the energy of his mind to this virtue? Well, I have not seen any one whose energy was not equal to it. It may be there are such, but I have never met with them.

"The faults of individuals are peculiar to their particular class and surroundings; and it is by observing their faults that one comes to understand the condition of their good feelings towards their fellows.

"One may hear the right way in the morning, and at evening die.

"The scholar who is intent upon learning the right way, and who is yet ashamed of poor attire and poor food, is not worthy of being discoursed with.

"The masterly man's attitude to the world is not exclusively this or that: whatsoever is right, to that he will be a party.

"The masterly man has an eye to virtue, the common man, to earthly things; the former has an eye to penalties for error—the latter, to favor.

"Where there is habitual going after gain, there is much ill-will.

"When there is ability in a ruler to govern a country by adhering to the Rules of Propriety, and by kindly condescension, what is wanted more? Where the ability to govern thus is wanting, what has such a ruler to do with the Rules of Propriety?

"One should not be greatly concerned at not being in office; but rather about the requirements in one's self for such a standing. Neither should one be so much concerned at being unknown; but rather with seeking to become worthy of being known."

Addressing his disciple Tsang Sin, the Master said, "Tsang Sin, the principles which I inculcate have one main idea upon which they all hang." "Aye, surely," he replied.

When the Master was gone out the other disciples asked what was the purport of this remark. Tsang's answer was, "The principles of our Master's teaching are these—whole-heartedness and kindly forbearance; these and nothing more."

Other observations of the Master:—

"Men of loftier mind manifest themselves in their equitable dealings; small-minded men in their going after gain.

"When you meet with men of worth, think how you may attain to their level; when you see others of an opposite character, look within, and examine yourself.

"A son, in ministering to his parents, may (on occasion) offer gentle remonstrances; when he sees that their will is not to heed such, he should nevertheless still continue to show them reverent respect, never obstinacy; and if he have to suffer, let him do so without murmuring.

"Whilst the parents are still living, he should not wander far; or, if a wanderer, he should at least have some fixed address.

"If for three years he do not veer from the principles of his father, he may be called a dutiful son.

“A son should not ignore the years of his parents. On the one hand, they may be a matter for rejoicing (that they have been so many), and on the other, for apprehension (that so few remain).

“People in olden times were loth to speak out, fearing the disgrace of not being themselves as good as their words.

“Those who keep within restraints are seldom losers.

“To be slow to speak, but prompt to act, is the desire of the ’superior man.’

“Virtue dwells not alone: she must have neighbors.”

An observation of Tsz-yu:—
“Officiousness, in the service of princes, leads to disgrace: among friends, to estrangement.”

BOOK V

A Disciple and the Golden Rule—Miscellaneous

The Master pronounced Kung-ye Ch'ang, a disciple, to be a marriageable person; for although lying bound in criminal fetters he had committed no crime. And he gave him his own daughter to wife.

Of Nan Yung, a disciple, he observed, that in a State where the government was well conducted he would not be passed over in its appointments, and in one where the government was ill conducted he would evade punishment and disgrace. And he caused his elder brother's daughter to be given in marriage to him.

Of Tsz-tsien, a disciple, he remarked, "A superior man indeed is the like of him! But had there been none of superior quality in Lu, how should this man have attained to this excellence?"

Tsz-kung asked, "What of me, then?" "You," replied the Master—"You are a receptacle." "Of what sort?" said he. "One for high and sacred use," was the answer.

Some one having observed of Yen Yung that he was good-natured towards others, but that he lacked the gift of ready speech, the Master said, "What need of that gift? To stand up before men and pour forth a stream of glib words is generally to make yourself obnoxious to them. I know not about his good-naturedness; but at any rate what need of that gift?"

When the Master proposed that Tsi-tiau K'ai should enter the government service, the latter replied, "I can scarcely credit it." The Master was gratified.

"Good principles are making no progress," once exclaimed the Master. "If I were to take a raft, and drift about on the sea, would Tsz-lu, I wonder, be my follower there?" That disciple was delighted at hearing the suggestion; whereupon the Master continued, "He surpasses me in his love of deeds of daring. But he does not in the least grasp the pith of my remark."

In reply to a question put to him by Mang Wu respecting Tsz-lu—as to whether he might be called good-natured towards others, the Master said, "I cannot tell"; but, on the question being put again, he answered, "Well, in an important State [10] he might be intrusted with the management of the military levies; but I cannot answer for his good nature."

"What say you then of Yen Yu?"

"As for Yen," he replied, "in a city of a thousand families, or in a secondary fief, [11] he might be charged with the governorship; but I cannot answer for his good-naturedness."

"Take Tsz-hwa, then; what of him?"

"Tsz-hwa," said he, "with a cincture girt upon him, standing as attendant at Court, might be charged with the addressing of visitors and guests; but as to his good-naturedness I cannot answer."

Addressing Tsz-kung, the Master said, "Which of the two is ahead of the other—yourself or Hwui?" "How shall I dare," he replied, "even to look at Hwui? Only let him hear one particular, and from that he knows ten; whereas I, if I hear one, may from it know two."

"You are not a match for him, I grant you," said the Master. "You are not his match."

Tsai Yu, a disciple, used to sleep in the daytime. Said the Master, "One may hardly carve rotten wood, or use a trowel to the wall of a manure-yard! In his case, what is the use of reprimand?

"My attitude towards a man in my first dealings with him," he added, "was to listen to his professions and to trust to his conduct. My attitude now is to listen to his professions, and to watch his conduct. My experience with Tsai Yu has led to this change.

"I have never seen," said the Master, "a man of inflexible firmness." Some one thereupon mentioned Shin Ch'ang, a disciple. "Ch'ang," said he, "is wanton; where do you get at his inflexibleness?"

Tsz-kung made the remark: "That which I do not wish others to put upon me, I also wish not to put upon others." "Nay," said the Master, "you have not got so far as that."

The same disciple once remarked, "There may be access so as to hear the Master's literary discourses, but when he is treating of human nature and the way of Heaven, there may not be such success."

Tsz-lu, after once hearing him upon some subject, and feeling himself as yet incompetent to carry into practice what he had heard, used to be apprehensive only lest he should hear the subject revived.

Tsz-kung asked how it was that Kung Wan had come to be so styled Wan (the talented). The Master's answer was, "Because, though a man of an active nature, he was yet fond of study, and he was not ashamed to stoop to put questions to his inferiors."

Respecting Tsz-ch'an,[12] the Master said that he had four of the essential qualities of the 'superior man':—in his own private walk he was humble-minded; in serving his superiors he was deferential; in his looking after the material welfare of the people he was generously kind; and in his exaction of public service from the latter he was just.

Speaking of Yen Ping, he said, "He was one who was happy in his mode of attaching men to him. However long the intercourse, he was always deferential to them."

Referring to Tsang Wan, he asked, "What is to be said of this man's discernment?—this man with his tortoise-house, with the pillar-heads and posts bedizened with scenes of hill and mere!"

Tsz-chang put a question relative to the chief Minister of Tsu, Tsz-wan. He said, "Three times he became chief Minister, and on none of these occasions did he betray any sign of exultation. Three times his ministry came to an end, and he showed no sign of chagrin. He used without fail to inform the new Minister as to the old mode of administration. What say you of him?"

"That he was a loyal man," said the Master.

"But was he a man of fellow-feeling?" said the disciple.

"Of that I am not sure," he answered; "how am I to get at that?"

The disciple went on to say:—"After the assassination of the prince of Ts'i by the officer Ts'ui, the latter's fellow-official Ch'in Wan, who had half a score teams of horses, gave up all, and turned his back upon him. On coming to another State, he observed, 'There are here characters somewhat like that of our minister Ts'ui,' and he turned his back upon them. Proceeding to a certain other State, he had occasion to make the same remark, and left. What say you of him?"

"That he was a pure-minded man," answered the Master.

"But was he a man of fellow-feeling?" urged the disciple.

"Of that I am not sure," he replied; "how am I to get at that?"

Ki Wan was one who thought three times over a thing before he acted. The Master hearing this of him, observed, "Twice would have been enough."

Of Ning Wu, the Master said that when matters went well in the State he used to have his wits about him: but when they went wrong, he lost them. His intelligence might be equalled, but not his witlessness!

Once, when the Master lived in the State of Ch'in, he exclaimed, "Let me get home again! Let me get home! My school-children [13] are wild and impetuous! Though they are somewhat accomplished, and perfect in one sense in their attainments, yet they know not how to make nice discriminations."

Of Peh-I and Shuh Ts'i he said, "By the fact of their not remembering old grievances, they gradually did away with resentment."

Of Wei-shang Kau he said, "Who calls him straightforward? A person once begged some vinegar of him, and he begged it from a neighbor, and then presented him with it!"

"Fine speech," said he, "and studied mien, and superfluous show of deference—of such things Tso-k'iu Ming was ashamed, I too am ashamed of such things. Also of hiding resentment felt towards an opponent and treating him as a friend—of this kind of thing he was ashamed, and so too am I."

Attended once by the two disciples Yen Yuen and Tsz-lu, he said, "Come now, why not tell me, each of you, what in your hearts you are really after?"

"I should like," said Tsz-lu, "for myself and my friends and associates, carriages and horses, and to be clad in light furs! nor would I mind much if they should become the worse for wear."

"And I should like," said Yen Yuen, "to live without boasting of my abilities, and without display of meritorious deeds."

Tsz-lu then said, "I should like, sir, to hear what your heart is set upon."

The Master replied, "It is this:—in regard to old people, to give them quiet and comfort; in regard to friends and associates, to be faithful to them; in regard to the young, to treat them with fostering affection and kindness."

On one occasion the Master exclaimed, "Ah, 'tis hopeless! I have not yet seen the man who can see his errors, so as inwardly to accuse himself."

"In a small cluster of houses there may well be," said he, "some whose integrity and sincerity may compare with mine; but I yield to none in point of love of learning."

[Footnote 10: Lit., a State of 1,000 war chariots.]

[Footnote 11: Lit., a House of 100 war chariots.]

[Footnote 12: A great statesman of Confucius's time.]

[Footnote 13: A familiar way of speaking of his disciples in their hearing.]

BOOK VI

More Characteristics—Wisdom—Philanthropy

Of Yen Yung, a disciple, the Master said, "Yung might indeed do for a prince!"

On being asked by this Yen Yung his opinion of a certain individual, the Master replied, "He is passable. Impetuous, though."

"But," argued the disciple, "if a man habituate himself to a reverent regard for duty—even while in his way of doing things he is impetuous—in the oversight of the people committed to his charge, is he not passable? If, on the other hand, he habituate himself to impetuosity of mind, and show it also in his way of doing things, is he not then over-impetuous?"

"You are right," said the Master.

When the Duke Ngai inquired which of the disciples were devoted to learning, Confucius answered him, "There was one Yen Hwui who loved it—a man whose angry feelings towards any particular person he did not suffer to visit upon another; a man who would never fall into the same error twice. Unfortunately his allotted time was short, and he died, and now his like is not to be found; I have never heard of one so devoted to learning."

While Tsz-hwa, a disciple, was away on a mission to Ts'i, the disciple Yen Yu, on behalf of his mother, applied for some grain. "Give her three pecks," said the Master. He applied for more. "Give her eight, then." Yen gave her fifty times that amount. The Master said, "When Tsz-hwa went on that journey to Ts'i, he had well-fed steeds yoked to his carriage, and was arrayed in light furs. I have learnt that the 'superior man' should help those whose needs are urgent, not help the rich to be more rich."

When Yuen Sz became prefect under him, he gave him nine hundred measures of grain, but the prefect declined to accept them.[14] "You must not," said the Master. "May they not be of use to the villages and hamlets around you?"

Speaking of Yen Yung again, the Master said, "If the offspring of a speckled ox be red in color, and horned, even though men may not wish to take it for sacrifice, would the spirits of the hills and streams reject it?"

Adverting to Hwui again, he said, "For three months there would not be in his breast one thought recalcitrant against his feeling of good-will towards his fellow-men. The others may attain to this for a day or for a month, but there they end."

When asked by Ki K'ang whether Tsz-lu was fit to serve the government, the Master replied, "Tsz-lu is a man of decision: what should prevent him from serving the government?"

Asked the same question respecting Tsz-kung and Yen Yu he answered similarly, pronouncing Tsz-kung to be a man of perspicacity, and Yen Yu to be one versed in the polite arts.

When the head of the Ki family sent for Min Tsz-k'ien to make him governor of the town of Pi, that disciple said, "Politely decline for me. If the offer is renewed, then indeed I shall feel myself obliged to go and live on the further bank of the Wan."

Peh-niu had fallen ill, and the Master was inquiring after him. Taking hold of his hand held out from the window, he said, "It is taking him off! Alas, his appointed time has come! Such a man, and to have such an illness!"

Of Hwui, again: "A right worthy man indeed was he! With his simple wooden dish of rice, and his one gourd-basin of drink, away in his poor back lane, in a condition too grievous for others to have endured, he never allowed his cheery spirits to droop. Aye, a right worthy soul was he!"

"It is not," Yen Yu once apologized, "that I do not take pleasure in your doctrines; it is that I am not strong enough." The Master rejoined, "It is when those who are not strong enough have made some moderate amount of progress that they fail and give up; but you are now drawing your own line for yourself."

Addressing Tsz-hia, the Master said, "Let your scholarship be that of gentlemen, and not like that of common men."

When Tsz-yu became governor of Wu-shing, the Master said to him, "Do you find good men about you?" The reply was, "There is Tan-t'ai Mieh-ming, who when walking eschews by-paths, and who, unless there be some public function, never approaches my private residence."

"Mang Chi-fan," said the Master, "is no sounder of his own praises. During a stampede he was in the rear, and as they were about to enter the city gate he whipped up his horses, and said, 'Twas not my daring made me lag behind. My horses would not go.'"

Obiter dicta of the Master:—

"Whoever has not the glib utterance of the priest T'o, as well as the handsomeness of Prince Chau of Sung, will find it hard to keep out of harm's way in the present age.

"Who can go out but by that door? Why walks no one by these guiding principles?

"Where plain naturalness is more in evidence than polish, we have—the man from the country. Where polish is more in evidence than naturalness, we have—the town scribe. It is when naturalness and polish are equally evident that we have the ideal man.

"The life of a man is—his rectitude. Life without it—such may you have the good fortune to avoid!

"They who know it are not as those who love it, nor they who love it as those who rejoice in it—that is, have the fruition of their love for it.

"To the average man, and those above the average, it is possible to discourse on higher subjects; to those from the average downwards, it is not possible."

Fan Ch'i put a query about wisdom. The Master replied, "To labor for the promoting of righteous conduct among the people of the land; to be serious in regard to spiritual beings, and to hold aloof from them;—this may be called wisdom."

To a further query, about philanthropy, he replied, "Those who possess that virtue find difficulty with it at first, success later.

"Men of practical knowledge," he said, "find their gratification among the rivers of the lowland, men of sympathetic social feeling find theirs among the hills. The former are active and bustling, the latter calm and quiet. The former take their day of pleasure, the latter look to length of days."

Alluding to the States of Ts'i and Lu, he observed, that Ts'i, by one change, might attain to the condition of Lu; and that Lu, by one change, might attain to good government.

An exclamation of the Master (satirizing the times, when old terms relating to government were still used while bereft of their old meaning):—"A quart, and not a quart! *quart*, indeed! *quart*, indeed!"

Tsai Wo, a disciple, put a query. Said he, "Suppose a philanthropic person were told, 'There's a fellow-creature down in the well!' Would he go down after him?"

"Why should he really do so?" answered the Master. "The good man or, a superior man might be induced to go, but not to go down. He may be misled, but not befooled."

"The superior man," said he, "with his wide study of books, and hedging himself round by the Rules of Propriety, is not surely, after all that, capable of overstepping his bounds."

Once when the Master had had an interview with Nan-tsz, which had scandalized his disciple Tsz-lu, he uttered the solemn adjuration, "If I have done aught amiss, may Heaven reject me! may Heaven reject me!"

"How far-reaching," said he, "is the moral excellence that flows from the Constant Mean! [15] It has for a long time been rare among the people."

Tsz-kung said, "Suppose the case of one who confers benefits far and wide upon the people, and who can, in so doing, make his bounty universally felt—how would you speak of him? Might he be called philanthropic?"

The Master exclaimed, "What a work for philanthropy! He would require indeed to be a sage! He would put into shade even Yau and Shun!—Well, a philanthropic person, desiring for himself a firm footing, is led on to give one to others; desiring for himself an enlightened perception of things, he is led on to help others to be similarly enlightened. If one could take an illustration coming closer home to us than yours, that might be made the starting-point for speaking about philanthropy."

[Footnote 14: At this time Confucius was Criminal Judge in his native State of Lu. Yuen Sz had been a disciple. The commentators add that this was the officer's proper salary, and that he did wrong to refuse it.]

[Footnote 15: The doctrine afterwards known by that name, and which gave its title to a Confucian treatise.]

BOOK VII

Characteristics of Confucius—An Incident

Said the Master:—

"I, as a transmitter[16] and not an originator, and as one who believes in and loves the ancients, venture to compare myself with our old P'ang.

"What find you indeed in me?—a quiet brooder and memorizer; a student never satiated with learning; an unwearied monitor of others!

"The things which weigh heavily upon my mind are these—failure to improve in the virtues, failure in discussion of what is learnt, inability to walk according to knowledge received as to what is right and just, inability also to reform what has been amiss."

In his hours of recreation and refreshment the Master's manner was easy and unconstrained, affable and winning.

Once he exclaimed, "Alas! I must be getting very feeble; 'tis long since I have had a repetition of the dreams in which I used to see the Duke of Chow. [17]

"Concentrate the mind," said he, "upon the Good Way.

"Maintain firm hold upon Virtue.

"Rely upon Philanthropy.

"Find recreation in the Arts. [18]

"I have never withheld instruction from any, even from those who have come for it with the smallest offering.

"No subject do I broach, however, to those who have no eager desire to learn; no encouraging hint do I give to those who show no anxiety to speak out their ideas; nor have I anything more to say to those who, after I have made clear one corner of the subject, cannot from that give me the other three."

If the Master was taking a meal, and there were any in mourning beside him, he would not eat to the full.

On one day on which he had wept, on that day he would not sing.

Addressing his favorite disciple, he said, "To you only and myself it has been given to do this—to go when called to serve, and to go back into quiet retirement when released from office."

Tsz-lu, hearing the remark said, "But if, sir, you had the handling of the army of one of the greater States,[19] whom would you have associated with you in that case?"

The Master answered:—

"Not the one 'who'll rouse the tiger,'
Not the one 'who'll wade the Ho;'

not the man who can die with no regret. He must be one who should watch over affairs with apprehensive caution, a man fond of strategy, and of perfect skill and effectiveness in it."

As to wealth, he remarked, "If wealth were an object that I could go in quest of, I should do so even if I had to take a whip and do grooms' work. But seeing that it is not, I go after those objects for which I have a liking."

Among matters over which he exercised great caution were times of fasting, war, and sickness.

When he was in the State of Ts'i, and had heard the ancient Shau music, he lost all perception of the taste of his meat. "I had no idea," said he, "that music could have been brought to this pitch."

In the course of conversation Yen Yu said, "Does the Master take the part of the Prince of Wei?" "Ah yes!" said Tsz-kung, "I will go and ask him that."

On going in to him, that disciple began, "What sort of men were Peh-I and Shuh Ts'i?" "Worthies of the olden time," the Master replied. "Had they any feelings of resentment?" was the next question. "Their aim and object," he answered, "was that of doing the duty which every man owes to his fellows, and they succeeded in doing it;—what room further for feelings of resentment?" The questioner on coming out said, "The Master does not take his part."

"With a meal of coarse rice," said the Master, "and with water to drink, and my bent arm for my pillow—even thus I can find happiness. Riches and honors without righteousness are to me as fleeting clouds."

"Give me several years more to live," said he, "and after fifty years' study of the 'Book of Changes' I might come to be free from serious error."

The Master's regular subjects of discourse were the "Books of the Odes" and "History," and the up-keeping of the Rules of Propriety. On all of these he regularly discoursed.

The Duke of Shih questioned Tsz-lu about Confucius, and the latter did not answer.

Hearing of this, the Master said, "Why did you not say, He is a man with a mind so intent on his pursuits that he forgets his food, and finds such pleasure in them that he forgets his troubles, and does not know that old age is coming upon him?"

"As I came not into life with any knowledge of it," he said, "and as my likings are for what is old, I busy myself in seeking knowledge there."

Strange occurrences, exploits of strength, deeds of lawlessness, references to spiritual beings—such-like matters the Master avoided in conversation.

"Let there," he said, "be three men walking together: from that number I should be sure to find my instructors; for what is good in them I should choose out and follow, and what is not good I should modify."

On one occasion he exclaimed, "Heaven begat Virtue in me; what can man do unto me?"

To his disciples he once said, "Do you look upon me, my sons, as keeping anything secret from you? I hide nothing from you. I do nothing that is not manifest to your eyes, my disciples. That is so with me."

Four things there were which he kept in view in his teaching—scholarliness, conduct of life, honesty, faithfulness.

"It is not given to me," he said, "to meet with a sage; let me but behold a man of superior mind, and that will suffice. Neither is it given to me to meet with a good man; let me but see a man of constancy, and it will suffice. It is difficult for persons to have constancy, when they pretend to have that which they are destitute of, to be full when they are empty, to do things on a grand scale when their means are contracted!"

When the Master fished with hook and line, he did not also use a net. When out with his bow, he would never shoot at game in cover.

"Some there may be," said he, "who do things in ignorance of what they do. I am not of these. There is an alternative way of knowing things, *viz.*—to sift out the good from the many things one hears, and follow it; and to keep in memory the many things one sees."

Pupils from Hu-hiang were difficult to speak with. One youth came to interview the Master, and the disciples were in doubt whether he ought to have been seen. "Why so much ado," said the Master, "at my merely permitting his approach, and not rather at my allowing him to draw back? If a man have cleansed himself in order to come and see me, I receive him as such; but I do not undertake for what he will do when he goes away."

"Is the philanthropic spirit far to seek, indeed?" the Master exclaimed; "I wish for it, and it is with me!"

The Minister of Crime in the State of Ch'in asked Confucius whether Duke Ch'an, of Lu was acquainted with the Proprieties; and he answered, "Yes, he knows them."

When Confucius had withdrawn, the minister bowed to Wu-ma K'i, a disciple, and motioned to him to come forward. He said, "I have heard that superior men show no partiality; are they, too, then, partial? That prince took for his wife a lady of the Wu family, having the same surname as himself, and had her named 'Lady Tsz of Wu, the elder,' If he knows the Proprieties, then who does not?"

The disciple reported this to the Master, who thereupon remarked, "Well for me! If I err in any way, others are sure to know of it."

When the Master was in company with any one who sang, and who sang well, he must needs have the song over again, and after that would join in it.

"Although in letters," he said, "I may have none to compare with me, yet in my personification of the 'superior man' I have not as yet been successful."

"'A Sage and a Philanthropist?' How should I have the ambition?" said he. "All that I can well be called is this—An insatiable student, an unwearied teacher;—this, and no more."—"Exactly what we, your disciples, cannot by any learning manage to be," said Kung-si Hwa.

Once when the Master was seriously ill, Tsz-lu requested to be allowed to say prayers for him. "Are such available?" asked the Master. "Yes," said he; "and the Manual of Prayers says, 'Pray to the spirits above and to those here below,'"

"My praying has been going on a long while," said the Master.

"Lavish living," he said, "renders men disorderly; miserliness makes them hard. Better, however, the hard than the disorderly."

Again, "The man of superior mind is placidly composed; the small-minded man is in a constant state of perturbation."

The Master was gentle, yet could be severe; had an over-awing presence, yet was not violent; was deferential, yet easy.

[Footnote 16: In reference to his editing the six Classics of his time.]

[Footnote 17: This was one of his "beloved ancients," famous for what he did in helping to found the dynasty of Chow, a man of great political wisdom, a scholar also, and poet. It was the "dream" of Confucius's life to restore the country to the condition in which the Duke of Chow left it.]

[Footnote 18: These were six in number, *viz.*: Ceremonial, Music, Archery, Horsemanship, Language, and Calculation.]

[Footnote 19: Lit., three forces. Each force consisted of 12,500 men, and three of such forces were the equipment of a greater State.]

BOOK VIII

Sayings of Tsang—Sentences of the Master

Speaking of T'ai-pih the Master said that he might be pronounced a man of the highest moral excellence; for he allowed the empire to pass by him onwards to a third heir; while the people, in their ignorance of his motives, were unable to admire him for so doing.

"Without the Proprieties," said the Master, "we have these results: for deferential demeanor, a worried one; for calm attentiveness, awkward bashfulness; for manly conduct, disorderliness; for straightforwardness, perversity.

"When men of rank show genuine care for those nearest to them in blood, the people rise to the duty of neighborliness and sociability. And when old friendships among them are not allowed to fall off, there will be a cessation of underhand practices among the people."

The Scholar Tsang was once unwell, and calling his pupils to him he said to them, "Disclose to view my feet and my hands. What says the Ode?—

'Act as from a sense of danger,
 With precaution and with care,
As a yawning gulf o'erlooking,
 As on ice that scarce will bear,'

At all times, my children, I know how to keep myself free from bodily harm."

Again, during an illness of his, Mang King, an official, went to ask after him. The Scholar had some conversation with him, in the course of which he said—

"'Doleful the cries of a dying bird,
 Good the last words of a dying man,'

There are three points which a man of rank in the management of his duties should set store upon:—A lively manner and deportment, banishing both severity and laxity; a frank and open expression of countenance, allied closely with sincerity; and a tone in his utterances utterly free from any approach to vulgarity and impropriety. As to matters of bowls and dishes, leave such things to those who are charged with the care of them."

Another saying of the Scholar Tsang: "I once had a friend who, though he possessed ability, would go questioning men of none, and, though surrounded by numbers, would go with his questions to isolated individuals; who also, whatever he might have, appeared as if he were without it, and, with all his substantial acquirements, made as though his mind were a mere blank; and when insulted would not retaliate;—this was ever his way."

Again he said: "The man that is capable of being intrusted with the charge of a minor on the throne, and given authority over a large territory, and who, during the important term of his superintendence cannot be forced out of his position, is not such a 'superior man'? That he is, indeed."

Again:—"The learned official must not be without breadth and power of endurance: the burden is heavy, and the way is long.

"Suppose that he take his duty to his fellow-men as his peculiar burden, is that not indeed a heavy one? And since only with death it is done with, is not the way long?"

Sentences of the Master:—

"From the 'Book of Odes' we receive impulses; from the 'Book of the Rules,' stability; from the 'Book on Music,' refinement. [20]

"The people may be put into the way they should go, though they may not be put into the way of understanding it.

"The man who likes bravery, and yet groans under poverty, has mischief in him. So, too, has the misanthrope, groaning at any severity shown towards him.

"Even if a person were adorned with the gifts of the Duke of Chow, yet if he were proud and avaricious, all the rest of his qualities would not indeed be worth looking at.

"Not easily found is the man who, after three years' study, has failed to come upon some fruit of his toil.

"The really faithful lover of learning holds fast to the Good Way till death.

"He will not go into a State in which a downfall is imminent, nor take up his abode in one where disorder reigns. When the empire is well ordered he will show himself; when not, he will hide himself away. Under a good government it will be a disgrace to him if he remain in poverty and low estate; under a bad one, it would be equally disgraceful to him to hold riches and honors.

"If not occupying the office, devise not the policy.

"When the professor Chi began his duties, how grand the finale of the First of the Odes used to be! How it rang in one's ears!

"I cannot understand persons who are enthusiastic and yet not straightforward; nor those who are ignorant and yet not attentive; nor again those folks who are simple-minded and yet untrue.

"Learn, as if never overtaking your object, and yet as if apprehensive of losing it.

"How sublime was the handling of the empire by Shun and Yu!—it was as nothing to them!

"How great was Yau as a prince! Was he not sublime! Say that Heaven only is great, then was Yau alone after its pattern! How profound was he! The people could not find a name for him. How sublime in his achievements! How brilliant in his scholarly productions!"

Shun had for his ministers five men, by whom he ordered the empire.

King Wu (in his day) stated that he had ten men as assistants for the promotion of order.

With reference to these facts Confucius observed, "Ability is hard to find. Is it not so indeed? During the three years' interregnum between Yau and Shun there was more of it than in the interval before this present dynasty appeared. There were, at this latter period, one woman, and nine men only.

"When two-thirds of the empire were held by King Wan, he served with that portion the House of Yin. We speak of the virtue of the House of Chow; we may say, indeed, that it reached the pinnacle of excellence."

"As to Yu," added the Master, "I can find no flaw in him. Living on meagre food and drink; yet providing to the utmost in his filial offerings to the spirits of the dead! Dressing in coarse garments; yet most elegant when vested in his sacrificial apron and coronet! Dwelling in a poor palace; yet exhausting his energies over those boundary-ditches and watercourses! I can find no flaw in Yu."

[Footnote 20: Comparison of three of the Classics: the "Shi-King," the "Li Ki," and the "Yoh." The last is lost.]

BOOK IX

His Favorite Disciple's Opinion of Him

Topics on which the Master rarely spoke were—Advantage, and Destiny, and Duty of man to man.

A man of the village of Tah-hiang exclaimed of him, "A great man is Confucius!—a man of extensive learning, and yet in nothing has he quite made himself a name!"

The Master heard of this, and mentioning it to his disciples he said, "What then shall I take in hand? Shall I become a carriage driver, or an archer? Let me be a driver!"

"The sacrificial cap," he once said, "should, according to the Rules, be of linen; but in these days it is of pure silk. However, as it is economical, I do as all do.

"The Rule says, 'Make your bow when at the lower end of the hall'; but nowadays the bowing is done at the upper part. This is great freedom; and I, though I go in opposition to the crowd, bow when at the lower end."

The Master barred four words:—he would have no "shall's," no "must's," no "certainty's," no "I's."

Once, in the town of K'wang fearing that his life was going to be taken, the Master exclaimed, "King Wan is dead and gone; but is not '*wan*' [21] with you here? If Heaven be about to allow this '*wan*' to perish, then they who survive its decease will get no benefit from it. But so long as Heaven does not allow it to perish, what can the men of K'wang do to me?"

A high State official, after questioning Tsz-kung, said, "Your Master is a sage, then? How many and what varied abilities must be his!"

The disciple replied, "Certainly Heaven is allowing him full opportunities of becoming a sage, in addition to the fact that his abilities are many and varied."

When the Master heard of this he remarked, "Does that high official know me? In my early years my position in life was low, and hence my ability in many ways, though exercised in trifling matters. In the gentleman is there indeed such variety of ability? No."

From this, the disciple Lau used to say, "'Twas a saying of the Master: 'At a time when I was not called upon to use them, I acquired my proficiency in the polite arts.'"

"Am I, indeed," said the Master, "possessed of knowledge? I know nothing. Let a vulgar fellow come to me with a question—a man with an emptyish head—I may thrash out with him the matter from end to end, and exhaust myself in doing it!"

"Ah!" exclaimed he once, "the phoenix does not come! and no symbols issue from the river! May I not as well give up?"

Whenever the Master met with a person in mourning, or with one in full-dress cap and kirtle, or with a blind person, although they might be young persons, he would make a point of rising on their appearance, or, if crossing their path, would do so with quickened step!

Once Yen Yuen exclaimed with a sigh (with reference to the Master's doctrines), "If I look up to them, they are ever the higher; if I try to penetrate them, they are ever the harder; if I gaze at them as if before my eyes, lo, they are behind me!—Gradually and gently the Master with skill lures men on. By literary lore he gave me breadth; by the Rules of Propriety he narrowed me down. When I desire a respite, I find it impossible; and after I have exhausted my powers, there seems to be something standing straight up in front of me, and though I have the mind to make towards it I make no advance at all."

Once when the Master was seriously ill, Tsz-lu induced the other disciples to feign they were high officials acting in his service. During a respite from his malady the Master exclaimed, "Ah! how long has Tsz-lu's conduct been false? Whom should I delude, if I were to pretend to have officials under me, having none? Should I deceive Heaven? Besides, were I to die, I would rather die in the hands of yourselves, my disciples, than in the hands of officials. And though I should fail to have a grand funeral over me, I should hardly be left on my death on the public highway, should I?"

Tsz-kung once said to him, "Here is a fine gem. Would you guard it carefully in a casket and store it away, or seek a good price for it and sell it?" "Sell it, indeed," said the Master—"that would I; but I should wait for the bidder."

The Master protested he would "go and live among the nine wild tribes."

"A rude life," said some one;—"how could you put up with it?"

"What rudeness would there be," he replied, "if a 'superior man' was living in their midst?"

Once he remarked, "After I came back from Wei to Lu the music was put right, and each of the Festal Odes and Hymns was given its appropriate place and use."

"Ah! which one of these following," he asked on one occasion, "are to be found exemplified in me—proper service rendered to superiors when abroad; duty to father and elder brother when at home; duty that shrinks from no exertion when dear ones die; and keeping free from the confusing effects of wine?"

Standing once on the bank of a mountain stream, he said (musingly), "Like this are those that pass away—no cessation, day or night!"

Other sayings:—

"Take an illustration from the making of a hill. A simple basketful is wanting to complete it, and the work stops. So I stop short.

"Take an illustration from the levelling of the ground. Suppose again just one basketful is left, when the work has so progressed. There I desist!

"Ah! it was Hwui, was it not? who, when I had given him his lesson, was the unflagging one!

"Alas for Hwui! I saw him ever making progress. I never saw him stopping short.

"Blade, but no bloom—or else bloom, but no produce; aye, that is the way with some!

"Reverent regard is due to youth. How know we what difference there may be in them in the future from what they are now? Yet when they have reached the age of forty or fifty, and are still unknown in the world, then indeed they are no more worthy of such regard.

"Can any do otherwise than assent to words said to them by way of correction? Only let them reform by such advice, and it will then be reckoned valuable. Can any be other than pleased with words of gentle suasion? Only let them comply with them fully, and such also will be accounted valuable. With those who are pleased without so complying, and those who assent but do not reform, I can do nothing at all.

"Give prominent place to loyalty and sincerity.

"Have no associates in study who are not advanced somewhat like yourself.

"When you have erred, be not afraid to correct yourself.

"It may be possible to seize and carry off the chief commander of a large army, but not possible so to rob one poor fellow of his will.

"One who stands—clad in hempen robe, the worse for wear—among others clad in furs of fox and badger, and yet unabashed—'tis Tsz-lu, that, is it not?"

Tsz-lu used always to be humming over the lines—

"From envy and enmity free,
What deed doth he other than good?"

"How should such a rule of life," asked the Master, "be sufficient to make any one good?"

"When the year grows chilly, we know the pine and cypress are the last to fade.

"The wise escape doubt; the good-hearted, trouble; the bold, apprehension.

"Some may study side by side, and yet be asunder when they come to the logic of things. Some may go on together in this latter course, but be wide apart in the standards they reach in it. Some, again, may together reach the same standard, and yet be diverse in weight of character."

"The blossom is out on the cherry tree,
  With a flutter on every spray.
Dost think that my thoughts go not out to thee?
  Ah, why art thou far away!"

Commenting on these lines the Master said, "There can hardly have been much 'thought going out,' What does distance signify?"

[Footnote 21: "Wan" was the honorary appellation of the great sage and ruler, whose praise is in the "Shi-King" as one of the founders of the Chow dynasty, and the term represented civic talent and virtues, as distinct from Wu, the martial talent—the latter being the honorary title of his son and successor. "Wan" also often stands for literature and polite accomplishments. Here Confucius simply means, "If you kill me, you kill a sage."]

BOOK X

Confucius in Private and Official Life

In his own village, Confucius presented a somewhat plain and simple appearance, and looked unlike a man who possessed ability of speech.

But in the ancestral temple, and at Court, he spoke with the fluency and accuracy of a debater, but ever guardedly.

At Court, conversing with the lower order of great officials, he spoke somewhat firmly and directly; with those of the higher order his tone was somewhat more affable.

When the prince was present he was constrainedly reverent in his movements, and showed a proper degree of grave dignity in demeanor.

Whenever the prince summoned him to act as usher to the Court, his look would change somewhat, and he would make as though he were turning round to do obeisance.

He would salute those among whom he took up his position, using the right hand or the left, and holding the skirts of his robe in proper position before and behind. He would make his approaches with quick step, and with elbows evenly bent outwards.

When the visitor withdrew, he would not fail to report the execution of his commands, with the words, "The visitor no longer looks back."

When he entered the palace gate, it was with the body somewhat bent forward, almost as though he could not be admitted. When he stood still, this would never happen in the middle of the gateway; nor when moving about would he ever tread on the threshold. When passing the throne, his look would change somewhat, he would turn aside and make a sort of obeisance, and the words he spoke seemed as though he were deficient in utterance.

On going up the steps to the audience chamber, he would gather up with both hands the ends of his robe, and walk with his body bent somewhat forward, holding back his breath like one in whom respiration has ceased. On coming out, after descending one step his countenance would relax and assume an appearance of satisfaction. Arrived at the bottom, he would go forward with quick step, his elbows evenly bent outwards, back to his position, constrainedly reverent in every movement.

When holding the sceptre in his hand, his body would be somewhat bent forward, as if he were not equal to carrying it; wielding it now higher, as in a salutation, now lower, as in the presentation of a gift; his look would also be changed and appear awestruck; and his gait would seem retarded, as if he were obeying some restraining hand behind.

When he presented the gifts of ceremony, he would assume a placid expression of countenance. At the private interview he would be cordial and affable.

The good man would use no purple or violet colors for the facings of his dress. [22] Nor would he have red or orange color for his undress. [23] For the hot season he wore a singlet, of either coarse or fine texture, but would also feel bound to have an outer garment covering it. For his black robe he had lamb's wool; for his white one, fawn's fur; and for his yellow one, fox fur. His furred undress robe was longer, but the right sleeve was shortened. He would needs have his sleeping-dress one and a half times his own length. For ordinary home wear he used thick substantial fox or badger furs. When he left off mourning, he would wear all his girdle trinkets. His kirtle in front, when it was not needed for full cover, he must needs have cut down. He would never wear his (black) lamb's-wool, or a dark-colored cap, when he went on visits of condolence to mourners. [24] On the first day of the new moon, he must have on his Court dress and to Court. When observing his fasts, he made a point of having bright, shiny garments, made of linen. He must also at such times vary his food, and move his seat to another part of his dwelling-room.

As to his food, he never tired of rice so long as it was clean and pure, nor of hashed meats when finely minced. Rice spoiled by damp, and sour, he would not touch, nor tainted fish, nor bad meat, nor aught of a bad color or smell, nor aught overdone in cooking, nor aught out of season. Neither would he eat anything that was not properly cut, or that lacked its proper seasonings. Although there might be an abundance of meat before him, he would not allow a preponderance of it to rob the rice of its beneficial effect in nutrition. Only in the matter of wine did he set himself no limit, yet he never drank so much as to confuse himself. Tradesmen's wines, and dried meats from the market, he would not touch. Ginger he would never have removed from the table during a meal. He was not a great eater. Meat from the sacrifices at the prince's temple he would never put aside till the following day. The meat of his own offerings he would never give out after three days' keeping, for after that time none were to eat it.

At his meals he would not enter into discussions; and when reposing (afterwards) he would not utter a word.

Even should his meal consist only of coarse rice and vegetable broth or melons, he would make an offering, and never fail to do so religiously.

He would never sit on a mat that was not straight.

After a feast among his villagers, he would wait before going away until the old men had left.

When the village people were exorcising the pests, he would put on his Court robes and stand on the steps of his hall to receive them.

When he was sending a message of inquiry to a person in another State, he would bow twice on seeing the messenger off.

Ki K'ang once sent him a present of some medicine. He bowed, and received it; but remarked, "Until I am quite sure of its properties I must not venture to taste it."

Once when the stabling was destroyed by fire, he withdrew from the Court, and asked, "Is any person injured? "—without inquiring as to the horses.

Whenever the prince sent him a present of food, he was particular to set his mat in proper order, and would be the first one to taste it. If the prince's present was one of raw meat, he must needs have it cooked, and make an oblation of it. If the gift were a live animal, he would be sure to keep it and care for it.

When he was in waiting, and at a meal with the prince, the prince would make the offering,[25] and he (the Master) was the pregustator.

When unwell, and the prince came to see him, he would arrange his position so that his head inclined towards the east, would put over him his Court robes, and draw his girdle across them.

When summoned by order of the prince, he would start off without waiting for his horses to be put to.

On his entry into the Grand Temple, he inquired about everything connected with its usages.

If a friend died, and there were no near relatives to take him to, he would say, "Let him be buried from my house."

For a friend's gift—unless it consisted of meat that had been offered in sacrifice—he would not bow, even if it were a carriage and horses.

In repose he did not lie like one dead. In his home life he was not formal in his manner.

Whenever he met with a person in mourning, even though it were a familiar acquaintance, he would be certain to change his manner; and when he met with any one in full-dress cap, or with any blind person, he would also unfailingly put on a different look, even though he were himself in undress at the time.

In saluting any person wearing mourning he would bow forwards towards the front bar of his carriage; in the same manner he would also salute the bearer of a census-register.

When a sumptuous banquet was spread before him, a different expression would be sure to appear in his features, and he would rise up from his seat.

At a sudden thunder-clap, or when the wind grew furious, his look would also invariably be changed.

On getting into his car, he would never fail (first) to stand up erect, holding on by the strap. When in the car, he would never look about, nor speak hastily, nor bring one hand to the other.

"Let one but make a movement in his face,
And the bird will rise and seek some safer place."

Apropos of this, he said, "Here is a hen-pheasant from Shan Liang—and in season! and in season!" After Tsz-lu had got it prepared, he smelt it thrice, and then rose up from his seat.

[Footnote 22: Because, it is said, such colors were adopted in fasting and mourning.]

[Footnote 23: Because they did not belong to the five correct colors (viz. green, yellow, carnation, white, and black), and were affected more by females.]

[Footnote 24: Since white was, as it is still, the mourning color.]

[Footnote 25: The act of "grace," before eating.]

BOOK XI

Comparative Worth of His Disciples

"The first to make progress in the Proprieties and in Music," said the Master, "are plain countrymen; after them, the men of higher standing. If I had to employ any of them, I should stand by the former."

"Of those," said he, "who were about me when I was in the Ch'in and Ts'ai States, not one now is left to approach my door."

"As for Hwui," [26] said the Master, "he is not one to help me on: there is nothing I say but he is not well satisfied with."

"What a dutiful son was Min Tsz-k'ien!" he exclaimed. "No one finds occasion to differ from what his parents and brothers have said of him."

Nan Yung used to repeat three times over the lines in the Odes about the white sceptre. Confucius caused his own elder brother's daughter to be given in marriage to him.

When Ki K'ang inquired which of the disciples were fond of learning, Confucius answered him, "There was one Yen Hwui who was fond of it; but unfortunately his allotted time was short, and he died; and now his like is not to be found."

When Yen Yuen died, his father, Yen Lu, begged for the Master's carriage in order to get a shell for his coffin. "Ability or no ability," said the Master, "every father still speaks of 'my son.' When my own son Li died, and the coffin for him had no shell to it, I know I did not go on foot to get him one; but that was because I was, though retired, in the wake of the ministers, and could not therefore well do so."

On the death of Yen Yuen the Master exclaimed, "Ah me! Heaven is ruining me, Heaven is ruining me!"

On the same occasion, his wailing for that disciple becoming excessive, those who were about him said, "Sir, this is too much!"—"Too much?" said he; "if I am not to do so for him, then—for whom else?"

The disciples then wished for the deceased a grand funeral. The Master could not on his part consent to this. They nevertheless gave him one. Upon this he remarked, "He used to look upon me as if I were his father. I could never, however, look on him as a son. Twas not my mistake, but yours, my children."

Tsz-lu propounded a question about ministering to the spirits of the departed. The Master replied, "Where there is scarcely the ability to minister to living men, how shall there be ability to minister to the spirits?" On his venturing to put a question concerning death, he answered, "Where there is scarcely any knowledge about life, how shall there be any about death?"

The disciple Min was by his side, looking affable and bland; Tsz-lu also, looking careless and intrepid; and Yen Yu and Tsz-kung, firm and precise. The Master was cheery. "One like Tsz-lu there," said he, "does not come to a natural end."

Some persons in Lu were taking measures in regard to the Long Treasury House. Min Tsz-k'ien observed, "How if it were repaired on the old lines?" The Master upon this remarked, "This fellow is not a talker, but when he does speak he is bound to hit the mark!"

"There is Yu's harpsichord," exclaimed the Master—"what is it doing at my door?" On seeing, however, some disrespect shown to him by the other disciples, he added, "Yu has got as far as the top of the hall; only he has not yet entered the house."

Tsz-kung asked which was the worthier of the two—Tsz-chang or Tsz-hia. "The former," answered the Master, "goes beyond the mark; the latter falls short of it."

"So then Tsz-chang is the better of the two, is he?" said he.

"To go too far," he replied, "is about the same as to fall short."

The Chief of the Ki family was a wealthier man than the Duke of Chow had been, and yet Yen Yu gathered and hoarded for him, increasing his wealth more and more.

"He is no follower of mine," said the Master. "It would serve him right, my children, to sound the drum, and set upon him."

Characteristics of four disciples:—Tsz-kau was simple-minded; Tsang Si, a dullard; Tsz-chang, full of airs; Tsz-lu, rough.

"As to Hwui," said the Master, "he comes near to perfection, while frequently in great want. Tsz-kung does not submit to the appointments of Heaven; and yet his goods are increased;—he is often successful in his calculations."

Tsz-chang wanted to know some marks of the naturally Good Man.

"He does not walk in others' footprints," said the Master; "yet he does not get beyond the hall into the house."

Once the Master said, "Because we allow that a man's words have something genuine in them, are they necessarily those of a superior man? or words carrying only an outward semblance and show of gravity?"

Tsz-lu put a question about the practice of precepts one has heard. The Master's reply was, "In a case where there is a father or elder brother still left with you, how should you practise all you hear?"

When, however, the same question was put to him by Yen Yu, his reply was, "Yes; do so."

Kung-si Hwa animadverted upon this to the Master. "Tsz-lu asked you, sir," said he, "about the practice of what one has learnt, and you said, 'There may be a father or elder brother still alive'; but when Yen Yu asked the same question, you answered, 'Yes, do so.' I am at a loss to understand you, and venture to ask what you meant."

The Master replied, "Yen Yu backs out of his duties; therefore I push him on. Tsz-lu has forwardness enough for them both; therefore I hold him back."

On the occasion of that time of fear in K'wang, Yen Yuen having fallen behind, the Master said to him (afterwards), "I took it for granted you were a dead man." "How should I dare to die," said he, "while you, sir, still lived?"

On Ki Tsz-jen putting to him a question anent Tsz-lu and Yen Yu, as to whether they might be called "great ministers," the Master answered, "I had expected your question, sir, to be about something extraordinary, and lo! it is only about these two. Those whom we call 'great ministers' are such as serve their prince conscientiously, and who, when they cannot do so, retire. At present, as regards the two you ask about, they may be called 'qualified ministers.'"

"Well, are they then," he asked, "such as will follow their leader?"

"They would not follow him who should slay his father and his prince!" was the reply.

Through the intervention of Tsz-lu, Tsz-kau was being appointed governor of Pi.

"You are spoiling a good man's son," said the Master.

Tsz-lu rejoined, "But he will have the people and their superiors to gain experience from, and there will be the altars; what need to read books? He can become a student afterwards."

"Here is the reason for my hatred of glib-tongued people," said the Master.

On one occasion Tsz-lu, Tsang Sin, Yen Yu, and Kung-si Hwa were sitting near him. He said to them, "Though I may be a day older than you, do not (for the moment) regard me as such. While you are living this unoccupied life you are saying, 'We do not become known.' Now suppose some one got to know you, what then?"

Tsz-lu—first to speak—at once answered, "Give me a State of large size and armament, hemmed in and hampered by other larger States, the population augmented by armies and regiments, causing a dearth in it of food of all kinds; give me charge of that State, and in three years' time I should make a brave country of it, and let it know its place."

The Master smiled at him. "Yen," said he, "how would it be with you?"

"Give me," said Yen, "a territory of sixty or seventy li square, or of fifty or sixty square; put me in charge of that, and in three years I should make the people sufficiently prosperous. As regards their knowledge of ceremonial or music, I should wait for superior men to teach them that."

"And with you, Kung-si, how would it be?"

This disciple's reply was, "I have nothing to say about my capabilities for such matters; my wish is to learn. I should like to be a junior assistant, in dark robe and cap, at the services of the ancestral temple, and at the Grand Receptions of the Princes by the Sovereign."

"And with you, Tsang Sin?"

This disciple was strumming on his harpsichord, but now the twanging ceased, he turned from the instrument, rose to his feet, and answered thus: "Something different from the choice of these three." "What harm?" said the Master; "I want each one of you to tell me what his heart is set upon." "Well, then," said he, "give me—in the latter part of spring—dressed in full spring-tide attire—in company with five or six young fellows of twenty, [27] or six or seven lads under that age, to do the ablutions in the I stream, enjoy a breeze in the rain-dance, [28] and finish up with songs on the road home."

The Master drew in his breath, sighed, and exclaimed, "Ah, I take with you!"

The three other disciples having gone out, leaving Tsang Sin behind, the latter said, "What think you of the answers of those three?"—"Well, each told me what was uppermost in his mind," said the Master;—"simply that."

"Why did you smile at Tsz-lu, sir?"

"I smiled at him because to have the charge of a State requires due regard to the Rules of Propriety, and his words betrayed a lack of modesty."

"But Yen, then—he had a State in view, had he not?"

"I should like to be shown a territory such as he described which does not amount to a State."

"But had not Kung-si also a State in view?"

"What are ancestral temples and Grand Receptions, but for the feudal lords to take part in? If Kung-si were to become an unimportant assistant at these functions, who could become an important one?"

[Footnote 26: The men of virtuous life were Yen Yuen (Hwui), Min Tsz-k'ien, Yen Pihniu, and Chung-kung (Yen Yung); the speakers and debaters were Tsai Wo and Tsz-kung; the (capable) government servants were Yen Yu and Tsz-lu; the literary students, Tsz-yu and Tsz-hia.]

[Footnote 27: Lit., capped ones. At twenty they underwent the ceremony of capping, and were considered men.]

[Footnote 28: *I.e.*, before the altars, where offerings were placed with prayer for rain. A religious dance.]

BOOK XII

The Master's Answers—Philanthropy—Friendships

Yen Yuen was asking about man's proper regard for his fellow-man. The Master said to him, "Self-control, and a habit of falling back upon propriety, virtually effect it. Let these conditions be fulfilled for one day, and every one round will betake himself to the duty. Is it to begin in one's self, or think you, indeed! it is to begin in others?"

"I wanted you to be good enough," said Yen Yuen, "to give me a brief synopsis of it."

Then said the Master, "Without Propriety use not your eyes; without it use not your ears, nor your tongue, nor a limb of your body."

"I may be lacking in diligence," said Yen Yuen, "but with your favor I will endeavor to carry out this advice."

Chung-kung asked about man's proper regard for his fellows.

To him the Master replied thus: "When you go forth from your door, be as if you were meeting some guest of importance. When you are making use of the common people (for State purposes), be as if you were taking part in a great religious function. Do not set before others what you do not desire yourself. Let there be no resentful feelings against you when you are away in the country, and none when at home."

"I may lack diligence," said Chung-kung, "but with your favor I will endeavor to carry out this advice."

Sz-ma Niu asked the like question. The answer he received was this: "The words of the man who has a proper regard for his fellows are uttered with difficulty."

"'His words—uttered with difficulty?'" he echoed, in surprise. "Is that what is meant by proper regard for one's fellow-creatures?"

"Where there is difficulty in doing," the Master replied, "will there not be some difficulty in utterance?"

The same disciple put a question about the "superior man." "Superior men," he replied, "are free from trouble and apprehension."

"'Free from trouble and apprehension!'" said he. "Does that make them 'superior men'?"

The Master added, "Where there is found, upon introspection, to be no chronic disease, how shall there be any trouble? how shall there be any apprehension?"

The same disciple, being in trouble, remarked, "I am alone in having no brother, while all else have theirs—younger or elder."

Tsz-hia said to him, "I have heard this: 'Death and life have destined times; wealth and honors rest with Heaven. Let the superior man keep watch over himself without ceasing, showing deference to others, with propriety of manners—and all within the four seas will be his brethren. How should he be distressed for lack of brothers!'" [29]

Tsz-chang asked what sort of man might be termed "enlightened."

The Master replied, "That man with whom drenching slander and cutting calumny gain no currency may well be called enlightened. Ay, he with whom such things make no way may well be called enlightened in the extreme."

Tsz-kung put a question relative to government. In reply the Master mentioned three essentials:—sufficient food, sufficient armament, and the people's confidence.

"But," said the disciple, "if you cannot really have all three, and one has to be given up, which would you give up first?"

"The armament," he replied.

"And if you are obliged to give up one of the remaining two, which would it be?"

"The food," said he. "Death has been the portion of all men from of old. Without the people's trust nothing can stand."

Kih Tsz-shing once said, "Give me the inborn qualities of a gentleman, and I want no more. How are such to come from book-learning?"

Tsz-kung exclaimed, "Ah! sir, I regret to hear such words from you. A gentleman!—But 'a team of four can ne'er o'er-take the tongue!' Literary accomplishments are much the same as inborn qualities, and inborn qualities as literary accomplishments. A tiger's or leopard's skin without the hair might be a dog's or sheep's when so made bare."

Duke Ngai was consulting Yu Joh. Said he, "It is a year of dearth, and there is an insufficiency for Ways and Means—what am I to do?"

"Why not apply the Tithing Statute?" said the minister.

"But two tithings would not be enough for my purposes," said the duke; "what would be the good of applying the Statute?"

The minister replied, "So long as the people have enough left for themselves, who of them will allow their prince to be without enough? But—when the people have not enough, who will allow their prince all that he wants?"

Tsz-chang was asking how the standard of virtue was to be raised, and how to discern what was illusory or misleading. The Master's answer was, "Give a foremost place to honesty and faithfulness, and tread the path of righteousness, and you will raise the standard of virtue. As to discerning what is illusory, here is an example of an illusion:—Whom you love you wish to live; whom you hate you wish to die. To have wished the same person to live and also to be dead—there is an illusion for you."

Duke King of Ts'i consulted Confucius about government. His answer was, "Let a prince be a prince, and ministers be ministers; let fathers be fathers, and sons be sons."

"Good!" exclaimed the duke; "truly if a prince fail to be a prince, and ministers to be ministers, and if fathers be not fathers, and sons not sons, then, even though I may have my allowance of grain, should I ever be able to relish it?"

"The man to decide a cause with half a word," exclaimed the Master, "is Tsz-lu!"

Tsz-lu never let a night pass between promise and performance.

"In hearing causes, I am like other men," said the Master. "The great point is—to prevent litigation."

Tsz-chang having raised some question about government, the Master said to him, "In the settlement of its principles be unwearied; in its administration—see to that loyally."

"The man of wide research," said he, "who also restrains himself by the Rules of Propriety, is not likely to transgress."

Again, "The noble-minded man makes the most of others' good qualities, not the worst of their bad ones. Men of small mind do the reverse of this."

Ki K'ang was consulting him about the direction of public affairs. Confucius answered him, "A director should be himself correct. If you, sir, as a leader show correctness, who will dare not to be correct?"

Ki K'ang, being much troubled on account of robbers abroad, consulted Confucius on the matter. He received this reply: "If you, sir, were not covetous, neither would they steal, even were you to bribe them to do so."

Ki K'ang, when consulting Confucius about the government, said, "Suppose I were to put to death the disorderly for the better encouragement of the orderly—what say you to that?"

"Sir," replied Confucius, "in the administration of government why resort to capital punishment? Covet what is good, and the people will be good. The virtue of the noble-minded man is as the wind, and that of inferior men as grass; the grass must bend, when the wind blows upon it."

Tsz-chang asked how otherwise he would describe the learned official who might be termed influential.

"What, I wonder, do you mean by one who is influential?" said the Master.

"I mean," replied the disciple, "one who is sure to have a reputation throughout the country, as well as at home."

"That," said the Master, "is reputation, not influence. The influential man, then, if he be one who is genuinely straightforward and loves what is just and right, a discriminator of men's words, and an observer of their looks, and in honor careful to prefer others to himself—will certainly have influence, both throughout the country and at home. The man of mere reputation, on the other hand, who speciously affects philanthropy, though in his way of procedure he acts contrary to it, while yet quite evidently engrossed with that virtue—will certainly have reputation, both in the country and at home."

Fan Ch'i, strolling with him over the ground below the place of the rain-dance, said to him, "I venture to ask how to raise the standard of virtue, how to reform dissolute habits, and how to discern what is illusory?"

"Ah! a good question indeed!" he exclaimed. "Well, is not putting duty first, and success second, a way of raising the standard of virtue? And is not attacking the evil in one's self, and not the evil which is in others, a way of reforming dissolute habits? And as to illusions, is not one morning's fit of anger, causing a man to forget himself, and even involving in the consequences those who are near and dear to him—is not that an illusion?"

The same disciple asked him what was meant by "a right regard for one's fellow-creatures." He replied, "It is love to man."

Asked by him again what was meant by wisdom, he replied, "It is knowledge of man."

Fan Ch'i did not quite grasp his meaning.

The Master went on to say, "Lift up the straight, set aside the crooked, so can you make the crooked straight."

Fan Ch'i left him, and meeting with Tsz-hia he said, "I had an interview just now with the Master, and I asked him what wisdom was. In his answer he said, 'Lift up the straight, set aside the crooked, and so can you make the crooked straight.' What was his meaning?"

"Ah! words rich in meaning, those," said the other. "When Shun was emperor, and was selecting his men from among the multitude, he 'lifted up' Kau-yau; and men devoid of right feelings towards their kind went far away. And when T'ang was emperor, and chose out his men from the crowd, he 'lifted up' I-yin—with the same result."

Tsz-kung was consulting him about a friend. "Speak to him frankly, and respectfully," said the Master, "and gently lead him on. If you do not succeed, then stop; do not submit yourself to indignity."

The learned Tsang observed, "In the society of books the 'superior man' collects his friends; in the society of his friends he is furthering good-will among men."

[Footnote 29: From Confucius, it is generally thought.]

BOOK XIII

Answers on the Art of Governing—Consistency

Tsz-lu was asking about government. "Lead the way in it," said the Master, "and work hard at it."

Requested to say more, he added, "And do not tire of it."

Chung-kung, on being made first minister to the Chief of the Ki family, consulted the Master about government, and to him he said, "Let the heads of offices be heads. Excuse small faults. Promote men of sagacity and talent."

"But," he asked, "how am I to know the sagacious and talented, before promoting them?"

"Promote those whom you do know," said the Master.

"As to those of whom you are uncertain, will others omit to notice them?"

Tsz-lu said to the Master, "As the prince of Wei, sir, has been waiting for you to act for him in his government, what is it your intention to take in hand first?"

"One thing of necessity," he answered—"the rectification of terms."

"That!" exclaimed Tsz-lu. "How far away you are, sir! Why such rectification?"

"What a rustic you are, Tsz-lu!" rejoined the Master. "A gentleman would be a little reserved and reticent in matters which he does not understand. If terms be incorrect, language will be incongruous; and if language be incongruous, deeds will be imperfect. So, again, when deeds are imperfect, propriety and harmony cannot prevail, and when this is the case laws relating to crime will fail in their aim; and if these last so fail, the people will not know where to set hand or foot. Hence, a man of superior mind, certain first of his terms, is fitted to speak; and being certain of what he says can proceed upon it. In the language of such a person there is nothing heedlessly irregular—and that is the sum of the matter."

Fan Ch'i requested that he might learn something of husbandry. "For that." said the Master, "I am not equal to an old husbandman." Might he then learn something of gardening? he asked. "I am not equal to an old gardener." was the reply.

"A man of little mind, that!" said the Master, when Fan Ch'i had gone out. "Let a man who is set over the people love propriety, and they will not presume to be disrespectful. Let him be a lover of righteousness, and they will not presume to be aught but submissive. Let him love faithfulness and truth, and they will not presume not to lend him their hearty assistance. Ah, if all this only were so, the people from all sides would come to such a one, carrying their children on their backs. What need to turn his hand to husbandry?

"Though a man," said he, "could hum through the Odes—the three hundred—yet should show himself unskilled when given some administrative work to do for his country; though he might know much of that other lore, yet if, when sent on a mission to any quarter, he could answer no question personally and unaided, what after all is he good for?

"Let a leader," said he, "show rectitude in his own personal character, and even without directions from him things will go well. If he be not personally upright, his directions will not be complied with."

Once he made the remark, "The governments of Lu and of Wei are in brotherhood."

Of King, a son of the Duke of Wei, he observed that "he managed his household matters well. On his coming into possession, he thought, 'What a strange conglomeration!'—Coming to possess a little more, it was, 'Strange, such a result!' And when he became wealthy, 'Strange, such elegance!'"

The Master was on a journey to Wei, and Yen Yu was driving him. "What multitudes of people!" he exclaimed. Yen Yu asked him, "Seeing they are so numerous, what more would you do for them?"

"Enrich them," replied the Master.

"And after enriching them, what more would you do for them?"

"Instruct them."

"Were any one of our princes to employ me," he said, "after a twelvemonth I might have made some tolerable progress;"

Again, "How true is that saying, 'Let good men have the management of a country for a century, and they would be adequate to cope with evil-doers, and thus do away with capital punishments,'"

Again, "Suppose the ruler to possess true kingly qualities, then surely after one generation there would be good-will among men."

Again, "Let a ruler but see to his own rectitude, and what trouble will he then have in the work before him? If he be unable to rectify himself, how is he to rectify others?"

Once when Yen Yu was leaving the Court, the Master accosted him. "Why so late?" he asked. "Busy with legislation," Yen replied. "The details of it," suggested the Master; "had it been legislation, I should have been there to hear it, even though I am not in office."

Duke Ting asked if there were one sentence which, if acted upon, might have the effect of making a country prosperous.

Confucius answered, "A sentence could hardly be supposed to do so much as that. But there is a proverb people use which says, 'To play the prince is hard, to play the minister not easy.' Assuming that it is understood that 'to play the prince is hard,' would it not be probable that with that one sentence the country should be made to prosper?"

"Is there, then," he asked, "one sentence which, if acted upon, would have the effect of ruining a country?"

Confucius again replied, "A sentence could hardly be supposed to do so much as that. But there is a proverb men have which says, 'Not gladly would I play the prince, unless my words were ne'er withstood.' Assuming that the words were good, and that none withstood them, would not that also be good? But assuming that they were not good, and yet none withstood them, would it not be probable that with that one saying he would work his country's ruin?"

When the Duke of Sheh consulted him about government, he replied, "Where the near are gratified, the far will follow."

When Tsz-hia became governor of Kue-fu, and consulted him about government, he answered, "Do not wish for speedy results. Do not look at trivial advantages. If you wish for speedy results, they will not be far-reaching; and if you regard trivial advantages you will not successfully deal with important affairs."

The Duke of Sheh in a conversation with Confucius said, "There are some straightforward persons in my neighborhood. If a father has stolen a sheep, the son will give evidence against him."

"Straightforward people in my neighborhood are different from those," said Confucius. "The father will hold a thing secret on his son's behalf, and the son does the same for his father. They are on their way to becoming straightforward."

Fan Ch'i was asking him about duty to one's fellow-men. "Be courteous," he replied, "in your private sphere; be serious in any duty you take in hand to do; be leal-hearted in your intercourse with others. Even though you were to go amongst the wild tribes, it would not be right for you to neglect these duties."

In answer to Tsz-kung, who asked, "how he would characterize one who could fitly be called 'learned official,'" the Master said, "He may be so-called who in his private life is affected with a sense of his own unworthiness, and who, when sent on a mission to any quarter of the empire, would not disgrace his prince's commands."

"May I presume," said his questioner, "to ask what sort you would put next to such?"

"Him who is spoken of by his kinsmen as a dutiful son, and whom the folks of his neighborhood call' good brother.'"

"May I still venture to ask whom you would place next in order?"

"Such as are sure to be true to their word, and effective in their work—who are given to hammering, as it were, upon one note—of inferior calibre indeed, but fit enough, I think, to be ranked next."

"How would you describe those who are at present in the government service?"

"Ugh! mere peck and panier men!—not worth taking into the reckoning."

Once he remarked, "If I cannot get *via media* men to impart instruction to, then I must of course take the impetuous and undisciplined! The impetuous ones will at least go forward and lay hold on things; and the undisciplined have at least something in them which needs to be brought out."

"The Southerners," said he, "have the proverb, 'The man who sticks not to rule will never make a charm-worker or a medical man,' Good!—'Whoever is intermittent in his practise of virtue will live to be ashamed of it.' Without prognostication," he added, "that will indeed be so."

"The nobler-minded man," he remarked, "will be agreeable even when he disagrees; the small-minded man will agree and be disagreeable."

Tsz-kung was consulting him, and asked, "What say you of a person who was liked by all in his village?"

"That will scarcely do," he answered.

"What, then, if they all disliked him?"

"That, too," said he, "is scarcely enough. Better if he were liked by the good folk in the village, and disliked by the bad."

"The superior man," he once observed, "is easy to serve, but difficult to please. Try to please him by the adoption of wrong principles, and you will fail. Also, when such a one employs others, he uses them according to their capacity. The inferior man is, on the other hand, difficult to serve, but easy to please. Try to please him by the adoption of wrong principles, and you will succeed. And when he employs others he requires them to be fully prepared for everything."

Again, "The superior man can be high without being haughty. The inferior man can be haughty if not high."

"The firm, the unflinching, the plain and simple, the slow to speak," said he once, "are approximating towards their duty to their fellow-men."

Tsz-lu asked how he would characterize one who might fitly be called an educated gentleman. The master replied, "He who can properly be so-called will have in him a seriousness of purpose, a habit of controlling himself, and an agreeableness of manner: among his friends and associates the seriousness and the self-control, and among his brethren the agreeableness of manner."

"Let good and able men discipline the people for seven years," said the Master, "and after that they may do to go to war."

But, said he, "To lead an undisciplined people to war—that I call throwing them away."

BOOK XIV

Good and Bad Government—Miscellaneous Sayings

Yuen Sz asked what might be considered to bring shame on one.

"Pay," said the Master; "pay—ever looking to that, whether the country be well or badly governed."

"When imperiousness, boastfulness, resentments, and covetousness cease to prevail among the people, may it be considered that mutual good-will has been effected?" To this question the Master replied, "A hard thing overcome, it may be considered. But as to the mutual good-will—I cannot tell."

"Learned officials," said he, "who hanker after a home life, are not worthy of being esteemed as such."

Again, "In a country under good government, speak boldly, act boldly. When the land is ill-governed, though you act boldly, let your words be moderate."

Again, "Men of virtue will needs be men of words—will speak out—but men of words are not necessarily men of virtue. They who care for their fellow-men will needs be bold, but the bold may not necessarily be such as care for their fellow-men."

Nan-kung Kwoh, who was consulting Confucius, observed respecting I, the skilful archer, and Ngau, who could propel a boat on dry land, that neither of them died a natural death; while Yu and Tsih, who with their own hands had labored at husbandry, came to wield imperial sway.

The Master gave him no reply. But when the speaker had gone out he exclaimed, "A superior man, that! A man who values virtue, that!"

"There have been noble-minded men," said he, "who yet were wanting in philanthropy; but never has there been a small-minded man who had philanthropy in him."

He asked, "Can any one refuse to toil for those he loves? Can any one refuse to exhort, who is true-hearted?"

Speaking of the preparation of Government Notifications in his day he said, "P'i would draw up a rough sketch of what was to be said; the Shishuh then looked it carefully through and put it into proper shape; Tsz-yu next, who was master of the ceremonial of State intercourse, improved and adorned its phrases; and Tsz-ch'an of Tung-li added his scholarly embellishments thereto."

To some one who asked his opinion of the last-named, he said, "He was a kind-hearted man." Asked what he thought of Tsz-si, he exclaimed, "Alas for him! alas for him!"—Asked again about Kwan Chung, his answer was, "As to him, he once seized the town of P'in with its three hundred families from the Chief of the Pih clan, who, afterwards reduced to living upon coarse rice, with all his teeth gone, never uttered a word of complaint."

"It is no light thing," said he, "to endure poverty uncomplainingly; and a difficult thing to bear wealth without becoming arrogant."

Respecting Mang Kung-ch'oh, he said that, while he was fitted for something better than the post of chief officer in the Chau or Wei families, he was not competent to act as minister in small States like those of T'ang or Sieh.

Tsz-lu asked how he would describe a perfect man. He replied, "Let a man have the sagacity of Tsang Wu-chung, the freedom from covetousness of Kung-ch'oh, the boldness of Chwang of P'in, and the attainments in polite arts of Yen Yu; and gift him further with the graces taught by the 'Books of Rites' and 'Music'—then he may be considered a perfect man. But," said he, "what need of such in these days? The man that may be regarded as perfect now is the one who, seeing some advantage to himself, is mindful of righteousness; who, seeing danger, risks his life; and who, if bound by some covenant of long standing, never forgets its conditions as life goes on."

Respecting Kung-shuh Wan, the Master inquired of Kung-ming Kia, saying, "Is it true that your master never speaks, never laughs, never takes aught from others?"

"Those who told you that of him," said he, "have gone too far. My master speaks when there is occasion to do so, and men are not surfeited with his speaking. When there is occasion to be merry too, he will laugh, but men have never overmuch of his laughing. And whenever it is just and right to take things from others, he will take them, but never so as to allow men to think him burdensome." "Is that the case with him?" said the Master. "Can it be so?"

Respecting Tsang Wu-chung the Master said, "When he sought from Lu the appointment of a successor to him, and for this object held on to his possession of the fortified city of Fang—if you say he was not then using constraint towards his prince, I must refuse to believe it."

Duke Wan of Tsin he characterized as "artful but not upright"; and Duke Hwan of Ts'i as "upright but not artful."

Tsz-lu remarked, "When Duke Hwan caused his brother Kiu to be put to death, Shau Hwuh committed suicide, but Kwan Chung did not. I should say he was not a man who had much good-will in him—eh?"

The Master replied, "When Duke Hwan held a great gathering of the feudal lords, dispensing with military equipage, it was owing to Kwan Chung's energy that such an event was brought about. Match such good-will as that—match it if you can."

Tsz-kung then spoke up. "But was not Kwan Chung wanting in good-will? He could not give up his life when Duke Hwan caused his brother to be put to death. Besides, he became the duke's counsellor."

"And in acting as his counsellor put him at the head of all the feudal lords," said the Master, "and unified and reformed the whole empire; and the people, even to this day, reap benefit from what he did. Had it not been for him we should have been going about with locks unkempt and buttoning our jackets (like barbarians) on the left. Would you suppose that he should show the same sort of attachment as exists between a poor yokel and his one wife—that he would asphyxiate himself in some sewer, leaving no one the wiser?"

Kung-shuh Wan's steward, who became the high officer Sien, went up accompanied by Wan to the prince's hall of audience.

When Confucius heard of this he remarked, "He may well be esteemed a 'Wan,'"

The Master having made some reference to the lawless ways of Duke Ling of Wei, Ki K'ang said to him, "If he be like that, how is it he does not ruin his position?"

Confucius answered, "The Chung-shuh, Yu, is charged with the entertainment of visitors and strangers; the priest T'o has charge of the ancestral temple; and Wang-sun Kia has the control of the army and its divisions:—with men such as those, how should he come to ruin?"

He once remarked, "He who is unblushing in his words will with difficulty substantiate them."

Ch'in Shing had slain Duke Kien. Hearing of this, Confucius, after performing his ablutions, went to Court and announced the news to Duke Ngai, saying, "Ch'in Hang has slain his prince. May I request that you proceed against him?"

"Inform the Chiefs of the Three Families," said the duke.

Soliloquizing upon this, Confucius said, "Since he uses me to back his ministers, [30] I did not dare not to announce the matter to him; and now he says, 'Inform the Three Chiefs.'"

He went to the Three Chiefs and informed them, but nothing could be done. Whereupon again he said, "Since he uses me to back his ministers, I did not dare not to announce the matter."

Tsz-lu was questioning him as to how he should serve his prince. "Deceive him not, but reprove him," he answered.

"The minds of superior men," he observed, "trend upwards; those of inferior men trend downwards."

Again, "Students of old fixed their eyes upon themselves: now they learn with their eyes upon others."

Kue Pih-yuh despatched a man with a message to Confucius. Confucius gave him a seat, and among other inquiries he asked, "How is your master managing?" "My master," he replied, "has a great wish to be seldom at fault, and as yet he cannot manage it."

"What a messenger!" exclaimed he admiringly, when the man went out. "What a messenger!"

"When not occupying the office," was a remark of his, "devise not the policy."

The Learned Tsang used to say, "The thoughts of the 'superior man' do not wander from his own office."

"Superior men," said the Master, "are modest in their words, profuse in their deeds."

Again, "There are three attainments of the superior man which are beyond me—the being sympathetic without anxiety, wise without scepticism, brave without fear."

"Sir," said Tsz-kung, "that is what you say of yourself."

Whenever Tsz-kung drew comparisons from others, the Master would say, "Ah, how wise and great you must have become! Now I have no time to do that."

Again, "My great concern is, not that men do not know me, but that they cannot."

Again, "If a man refrain from making preparations against his being imposed upon, and from counting upon others' want of good faith towards him, while he is foremost to perceive what is passing—surely that is a wise and good man."

Wi-shang Mau accosted Confucius, saying, "Kiu, how comes it that you manage to go perching and roosting in this way? Is it not because you show yourself so smart a speaker, now?"

"I should not dare do that," said Confucius. "Tis that I am sick of men's immovableness and deafness to reason."

"In a well-bred horse," said he, "what one admires is not its speed, but its good points."

Some one asked, "What say you of the remark, 'Requite enmity with kindness'?"

"How then," he answered, "would you requite kindness? Requite enmity with straightforwardness, and kindness with kindness."

"Ah! no one knows me!" he once exclaimed.

"Sir," said Tsz-kung, "how comes it to pass that no one knows you?"

"While I murmur not against Heaven," continued the Master, "nor cavil at men; while I stoop to learn and aspire to penetrate into things that are high; yet 'tis Heaven alone knows what I am."

Liau, a kinsman of the duke, having laid a complaint against Tsz-lu before Ki K'ang, an officer came to Confucius to inform him of the fact, and he added, "My lord is certainly having his mind poisoned by his kinsman Liau, but through my influence perhaps we may yet manage to see him exposed in the marketplace or the Court."

"If right principles are to have their course, it is so destined," said the Master; "if they are not to have their course, it is so destined. What can Liau do against Destiny?"

"There are worthy men," said the Master, "fleeing from the world; some from their district; some from the sight of men's looks; some from the language they hear."

"The men who have risen from their posts and withdrawn in this manner are seven in number."

Tsz-lu, having lodged overnight in Shih-mun, was accosted by the gate-keeper in the morning. "Where from?" he asked. "From Confucius," Tsz-lu responded. "That is the man," said he, "who knows things are not up to the mark, and is making some ado about them, is it not?"

When the Master was in Wei, he was once pounding on the musical stone, when a man with a basket of straw crossed his threshold, and exclaimed, "Ah, there is a heart that feels! Aye, drub the stone!" After which he added, "How vulgar! how he hammers away on one note!—and no one knows him, and he gives up, and all is over!

Be it deep, our skirts we'll raise to the waist,
—Or shallow, then up to the knee,'"

"What determination!" said the Master. "Yet it was not hard to do."

Tsz-chang once said to him, "In the 'Book of the Annals' it is stated that while Kau-tsung was in the Mourning Shed he spent the three years without speaking. What is meant by that?"

"Why must you name Kau-tsung?" said the Master. "It was so with all other ancient sovereigns: when one of them died, the heads of every department agreed between themselves that they should give ear for three years to the Prime Minister."

"When their betters love the Rules, then the folk are easy tools," was a saying of the Master.

Tsz-lu having asked what made a "superior man," he answered, "Self-culture, with a view to becoming seriously-minded."

"Nothing more than that?" said he.

"Self-culture with a view to the greater satisfaction of others," added the Master.

"That, and yet no more?"

"Self-culture with a view to the greater satisfaction of all the clans and classes," he again added. "Self-culture for the sake of all—a result that, that would almost put Yau and Shun into the shade!"

To Yuen Jang, [31] who was sitting waiting for him in a squatting (disrespectful) posture, the Master delivered himself as follows: "The man who in his youth could show no humility or subordination, who in his prime misses his opportunity, and who when old age comes upon him will not die—that man is a miscreant." And he tapped him on the shin with his staff.

Some one asked about his attendant—a youth from the village of Kiueh—whether he was one who improved. He replied, "I note that he seats himself in the places reserved for his betters, and that when he is walking he keeps abreast with his seniors. He is not one of those who care for improvement: he wants to be a man all at once."

[Footnote 30: Confucius had now retired from office, and this incident occurred only two years before his death.]

[Footnote 31: It is a habit with the Chinese, when a number are out walking together, for the eldest to go first, the others pairing off according to their age. It is a custom much older than the time of Confucius.]

BOOK XV

Practical Wisdom—Reciprocity the Rule of Life

Duke Ling of Wei was consulting Confucius about army arrangements. His answer was, "Had you asked me about such things as temple requisites, I have learnt that business, but I have not yet studied military matters." And he followed up this reply by leaving on the following day.

After this, during his residence in the State of Ch'in, his followers, owing to a stoppage of food supply, became so weak and ill that not one of them could stand. Tsz-lu, with indignation pictured on his countenance, exclaimed, "And is a gentleman to suffer starvation?"

"A gentleman," replied the Master, "will endure it unmoved, but a common person breaks out into excesses under it."

Addressing Tsz-kung, the Master said, "You regard me as one who studies and stores up in his mind a multiplicity of things—do you not?"—"I do," he replied; "is it not so?"—"Not at all. I have one idea—one cord on which to string all."

To Tsz-lu he remarked, "They who know Virtue are rare."

"If you would know one who without effort ruled well, was not Shun such a one? What did he indeed do? He bore himself with reverent dignity and undeviatingly 'faced the south,' and that was all."

Tsz-chang was consulting him about making way in life. He answered, "Be true and honest in all you say, and seriously earnest in all you do, and then, even if your country be one inhabited by barbarians, South or North, you will make your way. If you do not show yourself thus in word and deed how should you succeed, even in your own district or neighborhood?—When you are afoot, let these two counsels be two companions preceding you, yourself viewing them from behind; when you drive, have them in view as on the yoke of your carriage. Then may you make your way."

Tsz-chang wrote them on the two ends of his cincture.

"Straight was the course of the Annalist Yu," said the Master—"aye, straight as an arrow flies; were the country well governed or ill governed, his was an arrow-like course.

"A man of masterly mind, too, is Kue Pih-yuh! When the land is being rightly governed he will serve; when it is under bad government he is apt to recoil, and brood."

"Not to speak to a man." said he, "to whom you ought to speak, is to lose your man; to speak to one to whom you ought not to speak is to lose your words. Those who are wise will not lose their man nor yet their words."

Again, "The scholar whose heart is in his work, and who is philanthropic, seeks not to gain a livelihood by any means that will do harm to his philanthropy. There have been men who have destroyed their own lives in the endeavor to bring that virtue in them to perfection."

Tsz-kung asked how to become philanthropic. The Master answered him thus: "A workman who wants to do his work well must first sharpen his tools. In whatever land you live, serve under some wise and good man among those in high office, and make friends with the more humane of its men of education."

Yen Yuen consulted him on the management of a country. He answered:—

"Go by the Hia Calendar. Have the State carriages like those of the Yin princes. Wear the Chow cap. For your music let that of Shun be used for the posturers. Put away the songs of Ch'ing, and remove far from you men of artful speech: the Ch'ing songs are immodest, and artful talkers are dangerous."

Other sayings of the Master:—

"They who care not for the morrow will the sooner have their sorrow.

"Ah, 'tis hopeless! I have not yet met with the man who loves Virtue as he loves Beauty.

"Was not Tsang Wan like one who surreptitiously came by the post he held? He knew the worth of Hwui of Liu-hia, and could not stand in his presence.

"Be generous yourself, and exact little from others; then you banish complaints.

"With one who does not come to me inquiring 'What of this?' and 'What of that?' I never can ask 'What of this?' and give him up.

"If a number of students are all day together, and in their conversation never approach the subject of righteousness, but are fond merely of giving currency to smart little sayings, they are difficult indeed to manage.

"When the 'superior man' regards righteousness as the thing material, gives operation to it according to the Rules of Propriety, lets it issue in humility, and become complete in sincerity—there indeed is your superior man!

"The trouble of the superior man will be his own want of ability: it will be no trouble to him that others do not know him.

"Such a man thinks it hard to end his days and leave a name to be no longer named.

"The superior man is exacting of himself; the common man is exacting of others.

"A superior man has self-respect, and does not strive; is sociable, yet no party man.

"He does not promote a man because of his words, or pass over the words because of the man."

Tsz-kung put to him the question, "Is there one word upon which the whole life may proceed?"

The Master replied, "Is not Reciprocity such a word?—what you do not yourself desire, do not put before others."

"So far as I have to do with others, whom do I over-censure? whom do I over-praise? If there be something in them that looks very praiseworthy, that something I put to the test. I would have the men of the present day to walk in the straight path whereby those of the Three Dynasties have walked.

"I have arrived as it were at the annalist's blank page.—Once he who had a horse would lend it to another to mount; now, alas! it is not so.

"Artful speech is the confusion of Virtue. Impatience over little things introduces confusion into great schemes.

"What is disliked by the masses needs inquiring into; so also does that which they have a preference for.

"A man may give breadth to his principles: it is not principles (in themselves) that give breadth to the man.

"Not to retract after committing an error may itself be called error.

"If I have passed the whole day without food and the whole night without sleep, occupied with my thoughts, it profits me nothing: I were better engaged in learning.

"The superior man deliberates upon how he may walk in truth, not upon what he may eat. The farmer may plough, and be on the way to want: the student learns, and is on his way to emolument. To live a right life is the concern of men of nobler minds: poverty gives them none.

"Whatsoever the intellect may attain to, unless the humanity within is powerful enough to keep guard over it, is assuredly lost, even though it be gained.

"If there be intellectual attainments, and the humanity within is powerful enough to keep guard over them, yet, unless (in a ruler) there be dignity in his rule, the people will fail to show him respect.

"Again, given the intellectual attainments, and humanity sufficient to keep watch over them, and also dignity in ruling, yet if his movements be not in accordance with the Rules of Propriety, he is not yet fully qualified.

"The superior man may not be conversant with petty details, and yet may have important matters put into his hands. The inferior man may not be charged with important matters, yet may be conversant with the petty details.

"Good-fellowship is more to men than fire and water. I have seen men stepping into fire and into water, and meeting with death thereby; I have not yet seen a man die from planting his steps in the path of good-fellowship.

"Rely upon good nature. 'Twill not allow precedence even to a teacher.

"The superior man is inflexibly upright, and takes not things upon trust.

"In serving your prince, make your service the serious concern, and let salary be a secondary matter.

"Where instruction is to be given, there must be no distinction of persons.

"Where men's methods are not identical, there can be no planning by one on behalf of another.

"In speaking, perspicuity is all that is needed."

When the blind music-master Mien paid him a visit, on his approaching the steps the Master called out "Steps," and on his coming to the mat, said "Mat." When all in the room were seated, the Master told him "So-and-so is here, so-and-so is here."

When the music-master had left, Tsz-chang said to him, "Is that the way to speak to the music-master?" "Well," he replied, "it is certainly the way to assist him."

BOOK XVI

Against Intestine Strife—Good and Bad Friendships

The Chief of the Ki family was about to make an onslaught upon the Chuen-yu domain.

Yen Yu and Tsz-lu in an interview with Confucius told him, "The Ki is about to have an affair with Chuen-yu."

"Yen," said Confucius, "does not the fault lie with you? The Chief of Chuen-yu in times past was appointed lord of the East Mung (mountain); besides, he dwells within the confines of your own State, and is an official of the State-worship; how can you think of making an onslaught upon him?"

"It is the wish of our Chief," said Yen Yu, "not the wish of either of us ministers."

Confucius said, "Yen, there is a sentence of Chau Jin which runs thus: 'Having made manifest their powers and taken their place in the official list, when they find themselves incompetent they resign; if they cannot be firm when danger threatens the government, nor lend support when it is reeling, of what use then shall they be as Assistants?'—Besides, you are wrong in what you said. When a rhinoceros or tiger breaks out of its cage—when a jewel or tortoise-shell ornament is damaged in its casket—whose fault is it?"

"But," said Yen Yu, "so far as Chuen-yu is concerned, it is now fortified, and it is close to Pi; and if he does not now take it, in another generation it will certainly be a trouble to his descendants."

"Yen!" exclaimed Confucius, "it is a painful thing to a superior man to have to desist from saying, 'My wish is so-and-so,' and to be obliged to make apologies. For my part, I have learnt this—that rulers of States and heads of Houses are not greatly concerned about their small following, but about the want of equilibrium in it—that they do not concern themselves about their becoming poor, but about the best means of living quietly and contentedly; for where equilibrium is preserved there will be no poverty, where there is harmony their following will not be small, and where there is quiet contentment there will be no decline nor fall. Now if that be the case, it follows that if men in outlying districts are not submissive, then a reform in education and morals will bring them to; and when they have been so won, then will you render them quiet and contented. At the present time you two are Assistants of your Chief; the people in the outlying districts are not submissive, and cannot be brought round. Your dominion is divided, prostrate, dispersed, cleft in pieces, and you as its guardians are powerless. And plans are being made for taking up arms against those who dwell within your own State. I am apprehensive that the sorrow of the Ki family is not to lie in Chuen-yu, but in those within their own screen."

"When the empire is well-ordered," said Confucius, "it is from the emperor that edicts regarding ceremonial, music, and expeditions to quell rebellion go forth. When it is being ill governed, such edicts emanate from the feudal lords; and when the latter is the case, it will be strange if in ten generations there is not a collapse. If they emanate merely from the high officials, it will be strange if the collapse do not come in five generations. When the State-edicts are in the hands of the subsidiary ministers, it will be strange if in three generations there is no collapse.

"When the empire is well-ordered, government is not left in the hands of high officials.

"When the empire is well-ordered, the common people will cease to discuss public matters."

"For five generations," he said, "the revenue has departed from the ducal household. Four generations ago the government fell into the hands of the high officials. Hence, alas! the straitened means of the descendants of the three Hwan families."

"There are," said he, "three kinds of friendships which are profitable, and three which are detrimental. To make friends with the upright, with the trustworthy, with the experienced, is to gain benefit; to make friends with the subtly perverse, with the artfully pliant, with the subtle in speech, is detrimental."

Again, "There are three kinds of pleasure which are profitable, and three which are detrimental. To take pleasure in going regularly through the various branches of Ceremonial and Music, in speaking of others' goodness, in having many worthy wise friends, is profitable. To take pleasure in wild bold pleasures, in idling carelessly about, in the too jovial accompaniments of feasting, is detrimental."

Again, "Three errors there be, into which they who wait upon their superior may fall:—(1) to speak before the opportunity comes to them to speak, which I call heedless haste; (2) refraining from speaking when the opportunity has come, which I call concealment; and (3) speaking, regardless of the mood he is in, which I call blindness."

Again, "Three things a superior should guard against:—(1) against the lusts of the flesh in his earlier years while the vital powers are not fully developed and fixed; (2) against the spirit of combativeness when he has come to the age of robust manhood and when the vital powers are matured and strong, and (3) against ambitiousness when old age has come on and the vital powers have become weak and decayed."

"Three things also such a man greatly reveres:—(1) the ordinances of Heaven, (2) great men, (3) words of sages. The inferior man knows not the ordinances of Heaven and therefore reveres them not, is unduly familiar in the presence of great men, and scoffs at the words of sages."

"They whose knowledge comes by birth are of all men the first in understanding; they to whom it comes by study are next; men of poor intellectual capacity, who yet study, may be added as a yet inferior class; and lowest of all are they who are poor in intellect and never learn."

"Nine things there are of which the superior man should be mindful:—to be clear in vision, quick in hearing, genial in expression, respectful in demeanor, true in word, serious in duty, inquiring in doubt, firmly self-controlled in anger, just and fair when the way to success opens out before him."

"Some have spoken of 'looking upon goodness as upon something beyond their reach,' and of 'looking upon evil as like plunging one's hands into scalding liquid';—I have seen the men, I have heard the sayings.

"Some, again, have talked of 'living in seclusion to work out their designs,' and of 'exercising themselves in righteous living in order to render their principles the more effective';—I have heard the sayings, I have not seen the men."

"Duke King of Ts'i had his thousand teams of four, yet on the day of his death the people had nothing to say of his goodness. Peh-I and Shuh-Ts'i starved at the foot of Shau-yang, and the people make mention of them to this day.

'E'en if not wealth thine object be,
'Tis all the same, thou'rt changed to me.'

"Is not this apropos in such cases?"

Tsz-k'in asked of Pih-yu, "Have you heard anything else peculiar from your father?"

"Not yet," said he. "Once, though, he was standing alone when I was hurrying past him over the vestibule, and he said, 'Are you studying the Odes?' 'Not yet,' I replied. 'If you do not learn the Odes,' said he, 'you will not have the wherewithal for conversing,' I turned away and studied the Odes. Another day, when he was again standing alone and I was hurrying past across the vestibule, he said to me, 'Are you learning the Rules of Propriety?' 'Not yet,' I replied. 'If you have not studied the Rules, you have nothing to stand upon,' said he. I turned away and studied the Rules.—These two things I have heard from him."

Tsz-k'in turned away, and in great glee exclaimed, "I asked one thing, and have got three. I have learnt something about the Odes, and about the Rules, and moreover I have learnt how the superior man will turn away his own son."

The wife of the ruler of a State is called by her husband "My helpmeet." She speaks of herself as "Your little handmaiden." The people of that State call her "The prince's helpmeet," but addressing persons of another State they speak of her as

“Our little princess.” When persons of another State name her they say also “Your prince’s helpmeet.”

BOOK XVII

The Master Induced to Take Office—Nature and Habit

Yang Ho was desirous of having an interview with Confucius, but on the latter's failing to go and see him, he sent a present of a pig to his house. Confucius went to return his acknowledgments for it at a time when he was not at home. They met, however, on the way.

He said to Confucius, "Come, I want a word with you. Can that man be said to have good-will towards his fellow-men who hugs and hides his own precious gifts and allows his country to go on in blind error?"

"He cannot," was the reply.

"And can he be said to be wise who, with a liking for taking part in the public service, is constantly letting slip his opportunities?"

"He cannot," was the reply again.

"And the days and months are passing; and the years do not wait for us."

"True," said Confucius; "I will take office."

It was a remark of the Master that while "by nature we approximate towards each other, by experience we go far asunder."

Again, "Only the supremely wise and the most deeply ignorant do not alter."

The Master once, on his arrival at Wu-shing, heard the sound of stringed instruments and singing. His face beamed with pleasure, and he said laughingly, "To kill a cock—why use an ox-knife?"

Tsz-yu, the governor, replied, "In former days, sir, I heard you say, 'Let the superior man learn right principles, and he will be loving to other men; let the ordinary person learn right principles, and he will be easily managed.'"

The Master (turning to his disciples) said, "Sirs, what he says is right: what I said just now was only in play."

Having received an invitation from Kung-shan Fuh-jau, who was in revolt against the government and was holding to his district of Pi, the Master showed an inclination to go.

Tsz-lu was averse to this, and said, "You can never go, that is certain; how should you feel you must go to that person?"

"Well," said the Master, "he who has invited me must surely not have done so without a sufficient reason! And if it should happen that my services were enlisted, I might create for him another East Chow—don't you think so?"

Tsz-chang asked Confucius about the virtue of philanthropy. His answer was, "It is the being able to put in practice five qualities, in any place under the sun."

"May I ask, please, what these are?" said the disciple.

"They are," he said, "dignity, indulgence, faithfulness, earnestness, kindness. If you show dignity you will not be mocked; if you are indulgent you will win the multitude; if faithful, men will place their trust in you; if earnest, you will do something meritorious; and if kind, you will be enabled to avail yourself amply of men's services."

Pih Hih sent the Master an invitation, and he showed an inclination to go.

Tsz-lu (seeing this) said to him, "In former days, sir, I have heard you say, 'A superior man will not enter the society of one who does not that which is good in matters concerning himself'; and this man is in revolt, with Chung-man in his possession; if you go to him, how will the case stand?"

"Yes," said the Master, "those are indeed my words; but is it not said, 'What is hard may be rubbed without being made thin,' and 'White may be stained without being made black'?—I am surely not a gourd! How am I to be strung up like that kind of thing—and live without means?"

"Tsz-lu," said the Master, "you have heard of the six words with their six obfuscations?"

"No," said he, "not so far."

"Sit down, and I will tell you them. They are these six virtues, cared for without care for any study about them:—philanthropy, wisdom, faithfulness, straightforwardness, courage, firmness. And the six obfuscations resulting from not liking to learn about them are, respectively, these:—fatuity, mental dissipation, mischievousness, perversity, insubordination, impetuosity."

"My children," said he once, "why does no one of you study the Odes?—They are adapted to rouse the mind, to assist observation, to make people sociable, to arouse virtuous indignation. They speak of duties near and far—the duty of ministering to a parent, the duty of serving one's prince; and it is from them that one becomes conversant with the names of many birds, and beasts, and plants, and trees."

To his son Pih-yu he said, "Study you the Odes of Chow and the South, and those of Shau and the South. The man who studies not these is, I should say, somewhat in the position of one who stands facing a wall!"

"'Etiquette demands it.' 'Etiquette demands it,' so people plead," said he; "but do not these hankerings after jewels and silks indeed demand it? Or it is, 'The study of Music requires it'—'Music requires it'; but do not these predilections for bells and drums require it?"

Again, "They who assume an outward appearance of severity, being inwardly weak, may be likened to low common men; nay, are they not somewhat like thieves that break through walls and steal?"

Again, "The plebeian kind of respect for piety is the very pest of virtue."

Again, "Listening on the road, and repeating in the lane—this is abandonment of virtue."

"Ah, the low-minded creatures!" he exclaimed. "How is it possible indeed to serve one's prince in their company? Before they have got what they wanted they are all anxiety to get it, and after they have got it they are all anxiety lest they should lose it; and while they are thus full of concern lest they should lose it, there is no length to which they will not go."

Again, "In olden times people had three moral infirmities; which, it may be, are now unknown. Ambitiousness in those olden days showed itself in momentary outburst; the ambitiousness of to-day runs riot. Austerity in those days had its sharp angles; in these it is irritable and perverse. Feebleness of intellect then was at least straightforward; in our day it is never aught but deceitful."

Again, "Rarely do we find mutual good feeling where there is fine speech and studied mien."

Again, "To me it is abhorrent that purple color should be made to detract from that of vermilion. Also that the Odes of Ch'ing should be allowed to introduce discord in connection with the music of the Festal Songs and Hymns. Also that sharp-whetted tongues should be permitted to subvert governments."

Once said he, "Would that I could dispense with speech!"

"Sir," said Tsz-kung, "if you were never to speak, what should your pupils have to hand down from you?"

"Does Heaven ever speak?" said the Master. "The four seasons come and go, and all creatures live and grow. Does Heaven indeed speak?"

Once Ju Pi desired an interview with Confucius, from which the latter excused himself on the score of ill-health; but while the attendant was passing out through the doorway with the message he took his lute and sang, in such a way as to let him hear him.

Tsai Wo questioned him respecting the three years' mourning, saying that one full twelve-month was a long time—that, if gentlemen were for three years to cease from observing rules of propriety, propriety must certainly suffer, and that if for three years they neglected music, music must certainly die out—and that seeing nature has taught us that when the old year's grain is finished the new has sprung up for us—seeing also that all the changes[32] in procuring fire by friction have been gone through in the four seasons—surely a twelve-month might suffice.

The Master asked him, "Would it be a satisfaction to you—that returning to better food, that putting on of fine clothes?"

"It would," said he.

"Then if you can be satisfied in so doing, do so. But to a gentleman, who is in mourning for a parent, the choicest food will not be palatable, nor will the listening to music be pleasant, nor will comforts of home make him happy in mind. Hence he does not do as you suggest. But if you are now happy in your mind, then do so."

Tsai Wo went out. And the Master went on to say, "It is want of human feeling in this man. After a child has lived three years it then breaks away from the tender nursing of its parents. And this three years' mourning is the customary mourning prevalent all over the empire. Can this man have enjoyed the three years of loving care from his parents?"

"Ah, it is difficult," said he, "to know what to make of those who are all day long cramming themselves with food and are without anything to apply their minds to! Are there no dice and chess players? Better, perhaps, join in that pursuit than do nothing at all!"

"Does a gentleman," asked Tsz-lu, "make much account of bravery?"

"Righteousness he counts higher," said the Master. "A gentleman who is brave without being just may become turbulent; while a common person who is brave and not just may end in becoming a highwayman."

Tsz-kung asked, "I suppose a gentleman will have his aversions as well as his likings?"

"Yes," replied the Master, "he will dislike those who talk much about other people's ill-deeds. He will dislike those who, when occupying inferior places, utter defamatory words against their superiors. He will dislike those who, though they may be brave, have no regard for propriety. And he will dislike those hastily decisive and venturesome spirits who are nevertheless so hampered by limited intellect."

"And you, too, Tsz-kung," he continued, "have your aversions, have you not?"

"I dislike," said he, "those plagiarists who wish to pass for wise persons. I dislike those people who wish their lack of humility to be taken for bravery. I dislike also those divulgers of secrets who think to be accounted straightforward."

"Of all others," said the Master, "women-servants and men-servants are the most difficult people to have the care of. Approach them in a familiar manner, and they take liberties; keep them at a distance, and they grumble."

Again, "When a man meets with odium at forty, he will do so to the end."

[Footnote 32: Different woods were adopted for this purpose at the various seasons.]

BOOK XVIII

Good Men in Seclusion—Duke of Chow to His Son

"In the reign of the last king of the Yin dynasty," Confucius I said, "there were three men of philanthropic spirit:—the viscount of Wei, who withdrew from him; the viscount of Ki, who became his bondsman; and Pi-kan, who reproved him and suffered death."

Hwui of Liu-hia, who filled the office of Chief Criminal Judge, was thrice dismissed. A person remarked to him, "Can you not yet bear to withdraw?" He replied, "If I act in a straightforward way in serving men, whither in these days should I go, where I should not be thrice dismissed? Were I to adopt crooked ways in their service, why need I leave the land where my parents dwell?"

Duke King of Ts'i remarked respecting his attitude towards Confucius, "If he is to be treated like the Chief of the Ki family, I cannot do it. I should treat him as somewhere between the Ki and Mang Chiefs.—I am old," he added, "and not competent to avail myself of him."

Confucius, hearing of this, went away.

The Ts'i officials presented to the Court of Lu a number of female musicians. Ki Hwan accepted them, and for three days no Court was held.

Confucius went away.

Tsieh-yu, the madman [33] of Ts'u, was once passing Confucius, singing as he went along. He sang—

"Ha, the phoenix! Ha, the phoenix!
How is Virtue lying prone!
Vain to chide for what is o'er,
Plan to meet what's yet in store.
Let alone! Let alone!
Risky now to serve a throne."

Confucius alighted, wishing to enter into conversation with him; but the man hurried along and left him, and he was therefore unable to get a word with him.

Ch'ang-tsue and Kieh-nih [34] were working together on some ploughed land. Confucius was passing by them, and sent Tsz-lu to ask where the ford was.

Ch'ang-tsue said, "Who is the person driving the carriage?"

"Confucius," answered Tsz-lu.

"He of Lu?" he asked.

"The same," said Tsz-lu.

"He knows then where the ford is," said he.

Tsz-lu then put his question to Kieh-nih; and the latter asked, "Who are you?"

Tsz-lu gave his name.

"You are a follower of Confucius of Lu, are you not?"

"You are right," he answered.

"Ah, as these waters rise and overflow their bounds," said he, "'tis so with all throughout the empire; and who is he that can alter the state of things? And you are a follower of a learned man who withdraws from his chief; had you not better be a follower of such as have forsaken the world?" And he went on with his harrowing, without stopping.

Tsz-lu went and informed his Master of all this. He was deeply touched, and said, "One cannot herd on equal terms with beasts and birds: if I am not to live among these human folk, then with whom else should I live? Only when the empire is well ordered shall I cease to take part in the work of reformation."

Tsz-lu was following the Master, but had dropped behind on the way, when he encountered an old man with a weed-basket slung on a staff over his shoulder. Tsz-lu inquired of him, "Have you seen my Master, sir?" Said the old man, "Who is your master?—you who never employ your four limbs in laborious work; you who do not know one from another of the five sorts of grain!" And he stuck his staff in the ground, and began his weeding.

Tsz-lu brought his hands together on his breast and stood still.

The old man kept Tsz-lu and lodged him for the night, killed a fowl and prepared some millet, entertained him, and brought his two sons out to see him.

On the morrow Tsz-lu went on his way, and told all this to the Master, who said, "He is a recluse," and sent Tsz-lu back to see him again. But by the time he got there he was gone.

Tsz-lu remarked upon this, "It is not right he should evade official duties. If he cannot allow any neglect of the terms on which elders and juniors should live together, how is it that he neglects to conform to what is proper as between prince and public servant? He wishes for himself personally a pure life, yet creates disorder in that more important relationship. When a gentleman undertakes public work, he will carry out the duties proper to it; and he knows beforehand that right principles may not win their way."

Among those who have retired from public life have been Peh-I and Shuh-Ts'i, Yu-chung, I-yih, Chu-chang, Hwui of Liuhia, and Shau-lien.

"Of these," said the Master, "Peh-I and Shuh-Ts'i may be characterized, I should say, as men who never declined from their high resolve nor soiled themselves by aught of disgrace.

"Of Hwui of Liu-hia and Shau-lien, if one may say that they did decline from high resolve, and that they did bring disgrace upon themselves, yet their words were consonant with established principles, and their action consonant with men's thoughts and wishes; and this is all that may be said of them.

"Of Yu-chung and I-yih, if it be said that when they retired into privacy they let loose their tongues, yet in their aim at personal purity of life they succeeded, and their defection was also successful in its influence.

"My own rule is different from any adopted by these: I will take no liberties, I will have no curtailing of my liberty."

The chief music-master went off to Ts'i. Kan, the conductor of the music at the second repast, went over to Ts'u. Liau, conductor at the third repast, went over to Ts'ai. And Kiueh, who conducted at the fourth, went to Ts'in.

Fang-shuh, the drummer, withdrew into the neighborhood of the Ho. Wu the tambourer went to the Han. And Yang the junior music-master, and Siang who played on the musical stone, went to the sea-coast.

Anciently the Duke of Chow, addressing his son the Duke of Lu, said, "A good man in high place is not indifferent about the members of his own family, and does not give occasion to the chief ministers to complain that they are not employed; nor without great cause will he set aside old friendships; nor does he seek for full equipment for every kind of service in any single man."

There were once eight officials during this Chow dynasty, who were four pairs of twins, all brothers—the eldest pair Tab and Kwoh, the next Tub and Hwuh, the third Ye and Hia, the youngest Sui and Kwa.

[Footnote 33: He only pretended to be mad, in order to escape being employed in the public service.]

[Footnote 34: Two worthies who had abandoned public life, owing to the state of the times.]

BOOK XIX

Teachings of Various Chief Disciples

"The learned official," said Tsz-chang, "who when he sees danger ahead will risk his very life, who when he sees a chance of success is mindful of what is just and proper, who in his religious acts is mindful of the duty of reverence, and when in mourning thinks of his loss, is indeed a fit and proper person for his place."

Again he said, "If a person hold to virtue but never advance in it, and if he have faith in right principles and do not build himself up in them, how can he be regarded either as having such, or as being without them?"

Tsz-hia's disciples asked Tsz-chang his views about intercourse with others. "What says your Master?" he rejoined. "He says," they replied, "'Associate with those who are qualified, and repel from you such as are not,'" Tsz-chang then said, "That is different from what I have learnt. A superior man esteems the worthy and wise, and bears with all. He makes much of the good and capable, and pities the incapable. Am I eminently worthy and wise?—who is there then among men whom I will not bear with? Am I not worthy and wise?—others will be minded to repel me: I have nothing to do with repelling them."

Sayings of Tsz-hia:—

"Even in inferior pursuits there must be something worthy of contemplation, but if carried to an extreme there is danger of fanaticism; hence the superior man does not engage in them.

"The student who daily recognizes how much he yet lacks, and as the months pass forgets not what he has succeeded in learning, may undoubtedly be called a lover of learning.

"Wide research and steadfast purpose, eager questioning and close reflection—all this tends to humanize a man.

"As workmen spend their time in their workshops for the perfecting of their work, so superior men apply their minds to study in order to make themselves thoroughly conversant with their subjects.

"When an inferior man does a wrong thing, he is sure to gloss it over.

"The superior man is seen in three different aspects:—look at him from a distance, he is imposing in appearance; approach him, he is gentle and warm-hearted; hear him speak, he is acute and strict.

"Let such a man have the people's confidence, and he will get much work out of them; so long, however, as he does not possess their confidence they will regard him as grinding them down.

"When confidence is reposed in him, he may then with impunity administer reproof; so long as it is not, he will be regarded as a detractor.

"Where there is no over-stepping of barriers in the practice of the higher virtues, there may be freedom to pass in and out in the practice of the lower ones."

Tsz-yu had said, "The pupils in the school of Tsz-hia are good enough at such things as sprinkling and scrubbing floors, answering calls and replying to questions from superiors, and advancing and retiring to and from such; but these things are only offshoots—as to the root of things they are nowhere. What is the use of all that?"

When this came to the ears of Tsz-hia, he said, "Ah! there he is mistaken. What does a master, in his methods of teaching, consider first in his precepts? And what does he account next, as that about which he may be indifferent? It is like as in the study of plants—classification by *differentiae*. How may a master play fast and loose in his methods of instruction? Would they not indeed be sages, who could take in at once the first principles and the final developments of things?"

Further observations of Tsz-hia:—

"In the public service devote what energy and time remain to study. After study devote what energy and time remain to the public service.

"As to the duties of mourning, let them cease when the grief is past.

"My friend Tsz-chang, although he has the ability to tackle hard things, has not yet the virtue of philanthropy."

The learned Tsang observed, "How loftily Tsz-chang bears himself! Difficult indeed along with him to practise philanthropy!"

Again he said, "I have heard this said by the Master, that 'though men may not exert themselves to the utmost in other duties, yet surely in the duty of mourning for their parents they will do so!'"

Again, "This also I have heard said by the Master: 'The filial piety of Mang Chwang in other respects might be equalled, but as manifested in his making no changes among his father's ministers, nor in his father's mode of government—that aspect of it could not easily be equalled.'"

Yang Fu, having been made senior Criminal Judge by the Chief of the Mang clan, consulted with the learned Tsang. The latter advised him as follows: "For a long time the Chiefs have failed in their government, and the people have become unsettled. When you arrive at the facts of their cases, do not rejoice at your success in that, but rather be sorry for them, and have pity upon them."

Tsz-kung once observed, "We speak of 'the iniquity of Chau'—but 'twas not so great as this. And so it is that the superior man is averse from settling in this sink, into which everything runs that is foul in the empire."

Again he said, "Faults in a superior man are like eclipses of the sun or moon: when he is guilty of a trespass men all see it; and when he is himself again, all look up to him."

Kung-sun Ch'an of Wei inquired of Tsz-kung how Confucius acquired his learning.

Tsz-kung replied, "The teachings of Wan and Wu have not yet fallen to the ground. They exist in men. Worthy and wise men have the more important of these stored up in their minds; and others, who are not such, store up the less important of them; and as no one is thus without the teachings of Wan and Wu, how should our Master not have learned? And moreover what permanent preceptor could he have?"

Shuh-sun Wu-shuh, addressing the high officials at the Court, remarked that Tsz-kung was a greater worthy than Confucius.

Tsz-fuh King-pih went and informed Tsz-kung of this remark.

Tsz-kung said, "Take by way of comparison the walls outside our houses. My wall is shoulder-high, and you may look over it and see what the house and its contents are worth. My Master's wall is tens of feet high, and unless you should effect an entrance by the door, you would fail to behold the beauty of the ancestral hall and the rich array of all its officers. And they who effect an entrance by the door, methinks, are few! Was it not, however, just like him—that remark of the Chief?"

Shuh-sun Wu-shuh had been casting a slur on the character of Confucius.

"No use doing that," said Tsz-kung; "he is irreproachable. The wisdom and worth of other men are little hills and mounds of earth: traversible. He is the sun, or the moon, impossible to reach and pass. And what harm, I ask, can a man do to the sun or the moon, by wishing to intercept himself from either? It all shows that he knows not how to gauge capacity."

Tsz-k'in, addressing Tsz-kung, said, "You depreciate yourself. Confucius is surely not a greater worthy than yourself."

Tsz-kung replied, "In the use of words one ought never to be incautious; because a gentleman for one single utterance of his is apt to be considered a wise man, and for a single utterance may be accounted unwise. No more might one think of attaining to the Master's perfections than think of going upstairs to Heaven! Were it ever his fortune to be at the head of the government of a country, then that which is spoken of as 'establishing the country' would be establishment indeed; he would be its guide and it would follow him, he would tranquillize it and it would render its willing homage: he would give forward impulses to it to which it would harmoniously respond. In his life he would be its glory, at his death there would be great lamentation. How indeed could such as he be equalled?"

BOOK XX

Extracts from the Book of History

The Emperor Yau said to Shun, "Ah, upon you, upon your person, lies the Heaven-appointed order of succession! Faithfully hold to it, without any deflection; for if within the four seas necessity and want befall the people, your own revenue will forever come to an end."

Shun also used the same language in handing down the appointment to Yu.

The Emperor T'ang in his prayer, said, "I, the child Li, presume to avail me of an ox of dusky hue, and presume to manifestly announce to Thee, O God, the most high and Sovereign Potentate, that to the transgressor I dare not grant forgiveness, nor yet keep in abeyance Thy ministers. Judgment rests in Thine heart, O God. Should we ourself transgress, may the guilt not be visited everywhere upon all. Should the people all transgress, be the guilt upon ourself!"

Chow possessed great gifts, by which the able and good were richly endowed.

"Although," said King Wu, "he is surrounded by his near relatives, they are not to be compared with men of humane spirit. The people are suffering wrongs, and the remedy rests with me—the one man."

After Wu had given diligent attention to the various weights and measures, examined the laws and regulations, and restored the degraded officials, good government everywhere ensued.

He caused ruined States to flourish again, reinstated intercepted heirs, and promoted to office men who had gone into retirement; and the hearts of the people throughout the empire drew towards him.

Among matters of prime consideration with him were these—food for the people, the duty of mourning, and sacrificial offerings to the departed.

He was liberal and large-hearted, and so won all hearts; true, and so was trusted by the people; energetic, and thus became a man of great achievements; just in his rule, and all were well content.

Tsz-chang in a conversation with Confucius asked, "What say you is essential for the proper conduct of government?"

The Master replied, "Let the ruler hold in high estimation the five excellences, and eschew the four evils; then may he conduct his government properly."

"And what call you the five excellences?" he was asked.

"They are," he said, "Bounty without extravagance; burdening without exciting discontent; desire without covetousness; dignity without haughtiness; show of majesty without fierceness."

"What mean you," asked Tsz-chang, "by bounty without extravagance?"

"Is it not this," he replied—"to make that which is of benefit to the people still more beneficial? When he selects for them such labors as it is possible for them to do, and exacts them, who will then complain? So when his desire is the virtue of humaneness, and he attains it, how shall he then be covetous? And if—whether he have to do with few or with many, with small or with great—he do not venture ever to be careless, is not this also to have dignity without haughtiness? And if—when properly vested in robe and cap, and showing dignity in his every look—his appearance be so imposing that the people look up to and stand in awe of him, is not this moreover to show majesty without fierceness?"

"What, then, do you call the four evils?" said Tsz-chang.

The answer here was, "Omitting to instruct the people and then inflicting capital punishment on them—which means cruel tyranny. Omitting to give them warning and yet looking for perfection in them—which means oppression. Being slow and late in issuing requisitions, and exacting strict punctuality in the returns—which means robbery. And likewise, in intercourse with men, to expend and to receive in a stingy manner—which is to act the part of a mere commissioner."

"None can be a superior man," said the Master, "who does not recognize the decrees of Heaven.

"None can have stability in him without a knowledge of the proprieties.

"None can know a man without knowing his utterances."

THE SAYINGS OF MENICUS

[Translated into English by James Legge_]

INTRODUCTION

A hundred years after the time of Confucius the Chinese nation seemed to have fallen back into their original condition of lawlessness and oppression. The King's power and authority was laughed to scorn, the people were pillaged by the feudal nobility, and famine reigned in many districts. The foundations of truth and social order seemed to be overthrown. There were teachers of immorality abroad, who published the old Epicurean doctrine, "Let us eat and drink, for to-morrow we die." This teaching was accompanied by a spirit of cold-blooded egotism which extinguished every spark of Confucian altruism. Even the pretended disciples of Confucius confused the precepts of the Master, and by stripping them of their narrow significance rendered them nugatory. It was at this point that Mang-tsze, "Mang the philosopher," arose. He was sturdy in bodily frame, vigorous in mind, profound in political sagacity and utterly fearless in denouncing the errors of his countrymen. He had been brought up among the disciples of Confucius, in whose province he was born B.C. 372, but he was much more active and aggressive, less a Mystic than a fanatic, in comparison! with his Master. He resolved on active measures in stemming the tendency of his day. He did indeed surround himself with a school of disciples, but instead of making a series of desultory travels, teaching in remote places and along the high-road, he went to the heart of the evil. He presented himself like a second John the Baptist at the courts of kings and princes, and there boldly denounced vice and misrule. It was not difficult for a Chinese scholar and teacher to find access to the highest of the land. The Chinese believed in the divine right of learning, just as they believed in the divine right of kings. Mang employed every weapon of persuasion in trying to combat heresy and oppression; alternately ridiculing and reproving: now appealing in a burst of moral enthusiasm, and now denouncing in terms of cutting sarcasm the abuses which after all he failed to check. The last prince whom he successfully confronted was the Marquis of Lu, who turned him carelessly away. He accepted this as the Divine sentence of his failure, "That I have not found in this marquis, a ruler who would hearken to me is an intimation of heaven." Henceforth he lived in retirement until his ninety-seventh year; but from his apparent failure sprang a practical success. His written teachings are amongst the most lively and epigrammatic works of Chinese literature, have done much to keep alive amongst his countrymen the spirit of Confucianism, and even Western readers may drink wisdom from this spring of Oriental lore. The following selections from his sayings well exhibit the spirit of his system of philosophy and morality.

E.W.

BOOK I

KING HWUY OF LEANG

Part I

Mencius went to see King Hwuy of Leang. [1] The king said, "Venerable Sir, since you have not counted it far to come here a distance of a thousand li, may I presume that you are likewise provided with counsels to profit my kingdom?" Mencius replied, "Why must your Majesty used that word 'profit'? What I am likewise provided with are counsels to benevolence and righteousness; and these are my only topics.

"If your Majesty say, 'What is to be done to profit my kingdom?' the great officers will say, 'What is to be done to profit our families?' and the inferior officers and the common people will say, 'What is to be done to profit our persons?' Superiors and inferiors will try to take the profit the one from the other, and the kingdom will be endangered. In the kingdom of ten thousand chariots, the murderer of his ruler will be the chief of a family of a thousand chariots. In the State of a thousand chariots, the murderer of his ruler will be the chief of a family of a hundred chariots. To have a thousand in ten thousand, and a hundred in a thousand, cannot be regarded as not a large allowance; but if righteousness be put last and profit first, they will not be satisfied without snatching all.

"There never was a man trained to benevolence who neglected his parents. There never was a man trained to righteousness who made his ruler an after consideration. Let your Majesty likewise make benevolence and righteousness your only themes—- Why must you speak of profit?"

When Mencius, another day, was seeing King Hwuy of Leang, the King went and stood with him by a pond, and, looking round on the wild geese and deer, large and small, said, "Do wise and good princes also take pleasure in these things?" Mencius replied, "Being wise and good, they then have pleasure in these things. If they are not wise and good, though they have these things, they do not find pleasure." It is said in the 'Book of Poetry':—

'When he planned the commencement of the Marvellous tower,
He planned it, and defined it,
And the people in crowds undertook the work,
And in no time completed it.
When he planned the commencement, he said, "Be not in a hurry."
But the people came as if they were his children.
The king was in the Marvellous park,
Where the does were lying down—
The does so sleek and fat;
With the white birds glistening.
The king was by the Marvellous pond;—
How full was it of fishes leaping about!'

King Wan used the strength of the people to make his tower and pond, and the people rejoiced to do the work, calling the tower 'the Marvellous Tower,' and the pond 'the Marvellous Pond,' and being glad that he had his deer, his fishes and turtles. The ancients caused their people to have pleasure as well as themselves, and therefore they could enjoy it.

"In the Declaration of T'ang it is said, 'O Sun, when wilt thou expire? We will die together with thee.' The people wished for Keeh's death, though they should die with him. Although he had his tower, his pond, birds and animals, how could he have pleasure alone?"

King Hwuy of Leang said, "Small as my virtue is, in the government of my kingdom, I do indeed exert my mind to the utmost. If the year be bad inside the Ho, I remove as many of the people as I can to the east of it, and convey grain to the country inside. If the year be bad on the east of the river, I act on the same plan. On examining the governmental methods of the neighboring kingdoms, I do not find there is any ruler who exerts his mind as I do. And yet the people of the neighboring kings do not decrease, nor do my people increase—how is this?"

Mencius replied, "Your Majesty loves war; allow me to take an illustration from war. The soldiers move forward at the sound of the drum; and when the edges of their weapons have been crossed, on one side, they throw away their buff coats, trail their weapons behind them, and run. Some run a hundred paces and then stop; some run fifty paces and stop. What would you think if these, because they had run but fifty paces, should laugh at those who ran a hundred paces?" The king said, "They cannot do so. They only did not run a hundred paces; but they also ran." Mencius said, "Since your Majesty knows this you have no ground to expect that your people will become more numerous than those of the neighboring kingdoms.

"If the seasons of husbandry be not interfered with, the grain will be more than can be eaten. If close nets are not allowed to enter the pools and ponds, the fish and turtles will be more than can be consumed. If the axes and bills enter the hill-forests only at the proper times, the wood will be more than can be used. When the grain and fish and turtles are more than can be eaten, and there is more wood than can be used, this enables the people to nourish their living and do all offices for their dead, without any feeling against any. But this condition, in which the people nourish their living, and do all offices to their dead without having any feeling against any, is the first step in the Royal way.

"Let mulberry trees be planted about the homesteads with their five acres, and persons of fifty years will be able to wear silk. In keeping fowls, pigs, dogs, and swine, let not their time of breeding be neglected, and persons of seventy years will be able to eat flesh. Let there not be taken away the time that is proper for the cultivation of the field allotment of a hundred acres, and the family of several mouths will not suffer from hunger. Let careful attention be paid to the teaching in the various schools, with repeated inculcation of the filial and fraternal duties, and gray-haired men will not be seen upon the roads, carrying burdens on their backs or on their heads. It has never been that the ruler of a State where these results were seen, persons of seventy wearing silk and eating flesh, and the black-haired people suffering neither from hunger nor cold, did not attain to the Royal dignity.

"Your dogs and swine eat the food of men, and you do not know to store up of the abundance. There are people dying from famine on the roads, and you do not know to issue your stores for their relief. When men die, you say, 'It is not owing to me; it is owing to the year,' In what does this differ from stabbing a man and killing him, and then saying, 'It was not I; it was the weapon'? Let your Majesty cease to lay the blame on the year and instantly the people, all under the sky, will come to you."

King Hwuy of Leang said, "I wish quietly to receive your instructions." Mencius replied, "Is there any difference between killing a man with a stick and with a sword?" "There is no difference," was the answer.

Mencius continued, "Is there any difference between doing it with a sword and with governmental measures?" "There is not," was the answer again.

Mencius then said, "In your stalls there are fat beasts; in your stables there are fat horses. But your people have the look of hunger, and in the fields there are those who have died of famine. This is leading on beasts to devour men. Beasts devour one another, and men hate them for doing so. When he who is called the parent of the people conducts his government so as to be chargeable with leading on beasts to devour men, where is that parental relation to the people? Chung-ne said, 'Was he not without posterity who first made wooden images to bury with the dead?' So he said, because that man made the semblances of men and used them for that purpose; what shall be thought of him who causes his people to die of hunger?"

King Hwuy of Leang said, "There was not in the kingdom a stronger State than Ts'in, as you, venerable Sir, know. But since it descended to me, on the east we were defeated by Ts'e, and then my eldest son perished; on the west we lost seven hundred li of territory to Ts'in; and on the south we have sustained disgrace at the hands of Ts'oo. I have brought shame on my departed predecessors, and wish on their account to wipe it away once for all. What course is to be pursued to accomplish this?"

Mencius replied, "With a territory only a hundred li square it has been possible to obtain the Royal dignity. If your Majesty will indeed dispense a benevolent government to the people, being sparing in the use of punishments and fines, and making the taxes and levies of produce light, so causing that the fields shall be ploughed deep, and the weeding well attended to, and that the able-bodied, during their days of leisure, shall cultivate their filial piety, fraternal duty, faithfulness, and truth, serving thereby, at home, their fathers and elder brothers, and, abroad, their elders and superiors, you will then have a people who can be employed with sticks which they have prepared to oppose the strong buff-coats and sharp weapons of the troops of Ts'in and Ts'oo.

"The rulers of those States rob their people of their time, so that they cannot plough and weed their fields in order to support their parents. Parents suffer from cold and hunger; elder and younger brothers, wives and children, are separated and scattered abroad. Those rulers drive their people into pitfalls or into the water; and your Majesty will go to punish them. In such a case, who will oppose your Majesty? In accordance with this is the saying, 'The benevolent has no enemy!' I beg your Majesty not to doubt what I said."

Mencius had an interview with King Seang[2] of Leang. When he came out he said to some persons, "When I looked at him from a distance, he did not appear like a ruler; when I drew near to him, I saw nothing venerable about him. Abruptly he asked me, 'How can the kingdom, all under the sky, be settled?' I replied, 'It will be settled by being united under one sway,'

"'Who can so unite it?' he asked.

"I replied, 'He who has no pleasure in killing men can so unite it.'

"'Who can give it to him?' he asked.

"I replied, 'All under heaven will give it to him. Does your Majesty know the way of the growing grain? During the seventh and eighth months, when drought prevails, the plants become dry. Then the clouds collect densely in the heavens, and send down torrents of rain, so that the grain erects itself as if by a shoot. When it does so, who can keep it back? Now among those who are shepherds of men throughout the kingdom, there is not one who does not find pleasure in killing men. If there were one who did not find pleasure in killing men, all the people under the sky would be looking towards him with outstretched necks. Such being indeed the case, the people would go to him as water flows downwards with a rush, which no one can repress."

King Seuen of Ts'e asked, saying, "May I be informed by you of the transactions of Hwan of Ts'e and Wan of Ts'in?"

Mencius replied, "There were none of the disciples of Chung-ne who spoke about the affairs of Hwan and Wan, and therefore they have not been transmitted to these after-ages; your servant has not heard of them. If you will have me speak, let it be about the principles of attaining to the Royal sway."

The king said, "Of what kind must his virtue be who can attain to the Royal sway?" Mencius said, "If he loves and protects the people, it is impossible to prevent him from attaining it."

The king said, "Is such an one as poor I competent to love and protect the people?" "Yes," was the reply. "From what do you know that I am competent to that?" "I have heard," said Mencius, "from Hoo Heih the following incident:—'The king,' said he, 'was sitting aloft in the hall, when some people appeared leading a bull past below it. The king saw it, and asked where the bull was going, and being answered that they were going to consecrate a bell with its blood, he said, "Let it go, I cannot bear its frightened appearance—as if it were an innocent person going to the place of death." They asked in reply whether, if they did so, they should omit the consecration of the bell, but the king said, "How can that be omitted? Change it for a sheep."' I do not know whether this incident occurred."

"It did," said the king, and Mencius replied, "The heart seen in this is sufficient to carry you to the Royal sway. The people all supposed that your Majesty grudged the animal, but your servant knows surely that it was your Majesty's not being able to bear the sight of the creature's distress which made you do as you did."

The king said, "You are right; and yet there really was an appearance of what the people imagined. But though Ts'e be narrow and small, how should I grudge a bull? Indeed it was because I could not bear its frightened appearance, as if it were an innocent person going to the place of death, that therefore I changed it for a sheep."

Mencius said, "Let not your Majesty deem it strange that the people should think you grudged the animal. When you changed a large one for a small, how should they know the true reason? If you felt pained by its being led without any guilt to the place of death, what was there to choose between a bull and a sheep?" The king laughed and said, "What really was my mind in the matter? I did not grudge the value of the bull, and yet I changed it for a sheep! There was reason in the people's saying that I grudged the creature."

Mencius said, "There is no harm in their saying so. It was an artifice of benevolence. You saw the bull, and had not seen the sheep. So is the superior man affected towards animals, that, having seen them alive, he cannot bear to see them die, and, having heard their dying cries, he cannot bear to eat their flesh. On this account he keeps away from his stalls and kitchen."

The king was pleased and said, "The Ode says,

'What other men have in their minds,
I can measure by reflection,'

This might be spoken of you, my Master. I indeed did the thing, but when I turned my thoughts inward and sought for it, I could not discover my own mind. When you, Master, spoke those words, the movements of compassion began to work in my mind. But how is it that this heart has in it what is equal to the attainment of the Royal sway?"

Mencius said, "Suppose a man were to make this statement to your Majesty, 'My strength is sufficient to lift three thousand catties, but is not sufficient to lift one feather; my eyesight is sharp enough to examine the point of an autumn hair, but I do not see a wagon-load of fagots,' would your Majesty allow what he said?" "No," was the king's remark, and Mencius proceeded, "Now here is kindness sufficient to reach to animals, and yet no benefits are extended from it to the people—how is this? is an exception to be made here? The truth is, the feather's not being lifted is because the strength was not used; the wagon-load of firewood's not being seen is because the eyesight was not used; and the people's not being loved and protected is because the kindness is not used. Therefore your Majesty's not attaining to the Royal sway is because you do not do it, and not because you are not able to do it."

The king asked, "How may the difference between him who does not do a thing and him who is not able to do it be graphically set forth?" Mencius replied, "In such a thing as taking the T'ae mountain under your arm, and leaping with it over the North Sea, if you say to people, 'I am not able to do it,' that is a real case of not being able. In such a matter as breaking off a branch from a tree at the order of a superior, if you say to people, 'I am not able to do it,' it is not a case of not being able to do it. And so your Majesty's not attaining to the Royal sway is not such a case as that of taking the T'ae mountain under your arm and leaping over the North Sea with it; but it is a case like that of breaking off a branch from a tree.

"Treat with reverence due to age the elders in your own family, so that those in the families of others shall be similarly treated; treat with the kindness due to youth the young in your own family, so that those in the families of others shall be similarly treated—do this and the kingdom may be made to go round in your palm. It is said in the 'Book of Poetry,'

'His example acted on his wife,
Extended to his brethren,
And was felt by all the clans and States;'

Telling us how King Wan simply took this kindly heart, and exercised it towards those parties. Therefore the carrying out of the feeling of kindness by a ruler will suffice for the love and protection of all within the four seas; and if he do not carry it out, he will not be able to protect his wife and children. The way in which the ancients came greatly to surpass other men was no other than this, that they carried out well what they did, so as to affect others. Now your kindness is sufficient to reach to animals, and yet no benefits are extended from it to the people. How is this? Is an exception to be made here?

"By weighing we know what things are light, and what heavy. By measuring we know what things are long, and what short. All things are so dealt with, and the mind requires specially to be so. I beg your Majesty to measure it.—Your Majesty collects your equipments of war, endangers your soldiers and officers and excites the resentment of the various princes—do these things cause you pleasure in your mind?"

The king said, "No. How should I derive pleasure from these things? My object in them is to seek for what I greatly desire."

Mencius said, "May I hear from you what it is that your Majesty greatly desires?" The king laughed, and did not speak. Mencius resumed, "Are you led to desire it because you have not enough of rich and sweet food for your mouth? or because you have not enough of light and warm clothing for your body? or because you have not enough of beautifully colored objects to satisfy your eyes? or because there are not voices and sounds enough to fill your ears? or because you have not enough of attendants and favorites to stand before you and receive your orders? Your Majesty's various officers are sufficient to supply you with all these things. How can your Majesty have such a desire on account of them?" "No," said the king, "my desire is not on account of them." Mencius observed, "Then what your Majesty greatly desires can be known. You desire to enlarge your territories, to have Ts'in and Ts'oo coming to your court, to rule the Middle States, and to attract to you the barbarous tribes that surround them. But to do what you do in order to seek for what you desire is like climbing a tree to seek for fish."

"Is it so bad as that?" said the king. "I apprehend it is worse," was the reply. "If you climb a tree to seek for fish, although you do not get the fish, you have no subsequent calamity. But if you do what you do in order to seek for what you desire, doing it even with all your heart, you will assuredly afterwards meet with calamities." The king said, "May I hear what they will be?" Mencius replied, "If the people of Tsow were fighting with the people of Ts'oo, which of them does your Majesty think would conquer?" "The people of Ts'oo would conquer," was the answer, and Mencius pursued, "So then, a small State cannot contend with a great, few cannot contend with many, nor can the weak contend with the strong. The territory within the seas would embrace nine divisions, each of a thousand li square. All Ts'e together is one of them. If with one part you try to subdue the other eight, what is the difference between that and Tsow's contending with Ts'oo? With the desire which you have, you must turn back to the proper course for its attainment.

"Now, if your Majesty will institute a government whose action shall all be benevolent, this will cause all the officers in the kingdom to wish to stand in your Majesty's court, the farmers all to wish to plough in your Majesty's fields, the merchants, both travelling and stationary, all to wish to store their goods in your Majesty's market-places, travellers and visitors all to wish to travel on your Majesty's roads, and all under heaven who feel aggrieved by their rulers to wish to come and complain to your Majesty. When they are so bent, who will be able to keep them back?"

The king said, "I am stupid and cannot advance to this. But I wish you, my Master, to assist my intentions. Teach me clearly, and although I am deficient in intelligence and vigor, I should like to try at least to institute such a government."

Mencius replied, "They are only men of education, who, without a certain livelihood, are able to maintain a fixed heart. As to the people, if they have not a certain livelihood, they will be found not to have a fixed heart. And if they have not a fixed heart, there is nothing which they will not do in the way of self-abandonment, of moral deflection, of depravity, and of wild license. When they have thus been involved in crime, to follow them up and punish them, is to entrap the people. How can such a thing as entrapping the people be done under the rule of a benevolent man?"

"Therefore, an intelligent ruler will regulate the livelihood of the people, so as to make sure that, above, they shall have sufficient wherewith to serve their parents, and below, sufficient wherewith to support their wives and children; that in good years they shall always be abundantly satisfied, and that in bad years they shall not be in danger of perishing. After this he may urge them, and they will proceed to what is good, for in this case the people will follow after that with readiness.

"But now the livelihood of the people is so regulated, that, above, they have not sufficient wherewith to serve their parents, and, below, they have not sufficient wherewith to support their wives and children; even in good years their lives are always embittered, and in bad years they are in danger of perishing. In such circumstances their only object is to escape from death, and they are afraid they will not succeed in doing so—what leisure have they to cultivate propriety and righteousness?

"If your Majesty wishes to carry out a benevolent government, why not turn back to what is the essential step to its attainment?

"Let mulberry trees be planted about the homesteads with their five acres, and persons of fifty years will be able to wear silk. In keeping fowls, pigs, dogs, and swine, let not their times of breeding be neglected, and persons of seventy years will be able to eat flesh. Let there not be taken away the time that is proper for the cultivation of the field-allotment of a hundred acres, and the family of eight mouths will not suffer from hunger. Let careful attention be paid to the teaching in the various schools, with repeated inculcation of the filial and fraternal duties, and gray-haired men will not be seen upon the roads, carrying burdens on their backs or on their heads. It has never been that the ruler of a State, where these results were seen, the old wearing silk and eating flesh, and the black-haired people suffering neither from hunger nor cold, did not attain to the Royal dignity."

[NOTE: *Books II, III, and IV are omitted*]

[Footnote 1: The title of this book in Chinese is—"King Hwuy of Leang; in chapters and sentences." Like the Books of the Confucian Analects, those of this work are headed by two or three words at or near the commencement of them. Each Book is divided into two parts. This arrangement was made by Chaou K'e, and to him are due also the divisions into chapters, and sentences, or paragraphs, containing, it may be, many sentences.]

[Footnote 2: Seang was the son of King Hwuy. The first year of his reign is supposed to be B.C. 317. Seang's name was Hih. As a posthumous epithet, Seang has various meanings: "Land-enlarger and Virtuous"; "Successful in Arms." The interview here recorded seems to have taken place immediately after Hih's accession, and Mencius, it is said, was so disappointed by it that he soon after left the country.]

THE SHI-KING

[*Metrical translation by James Legge*]

INTRODUCTION

The wisdom of Confucius as a social reformer, as a teacher and guide of the Chinese people, is shown in many ways. He not only gave them a code of personal deportment, providing them with rules for the etiquette and ceremony of life, but he instilled into them that profound spirit of domestic piety which is one of the strongest features in the Chinese character. He took measures to secure also the intellectual cultivation of his followers, and his Five Canons contain all the most ancient works of Chinese literature, in the departments of poetry, history, philosophy, and legislation. The Shi-King is a collection of Chinese poetry made by Confucius himself. This great anthology consists of more than three hundred pieces, covering the whole range of Chinese lyric poetry, the oldest of which dates some eighteen centuries before Christ, while the latest of the selections must have been written at the beginning of the sixth century before Christ. These poems are of the highest interest, and even nowadays may be read with delight by Europeans. The ballad and the hymn are among the earliest forms of national poetry, and the contents of the Shi-King naturally show specimens of lyric poetry of this sort. We find there not only hymns, but also ballads of a really fine and spirited character. Sometimes the poems celebrate the common pursuits, occupations, and incidents of life. They rise to the exaltation of the epithalamium, or of the vintage song; at other times they deal with sentiment and human conduct, being in the highest degree sententious and epigrammatic. We must give the credit to Confucius of having saved for us the literature of China, and of having set his people an example in preserving the monuments of a remote antiquity. While the literatures of ancient Greece and Rome have largely perished in the convulsions that followed the breaking up of the Roman empire in Europe, when the kingdom of China fell into disorder and decrepitude this one great teacher stepped forward to save the precious record of historic fact, philosophical thought, and of legislation as well as poetry, from being swept away by the deluge of revolution. Confucius showed his wisdom by the high value he set upon the poetry of his native land, and his name must be set side by side with that of the astute tyrant of Athens who collected the poems of Homer and preserved them as a precious heritage to the Greek world. Confucius has given us his opinion with regard to the poems of the Shi-King. No man, he says, is worth speaking to who has not mastered the poems of an anthology, the perusal of which elevates the mind and purifies it from all corrupt thoughts. Thanks to the work of modern scholarship, English readers can now verify this dictum for themselves.

E. W.

THE SHI-KING

PART I—LESSONS FROM THE STATES

BOOK I

THE ODES OF CHOW AND THE SOUTH

Celebrating the Virtue of King Wan's Bride

Hark! from the islet in the stream the voice
Of the fish-hawks that o'er their nests rejoice!
From them our thoughts to that young lady go,
Modest and virtuous, loth herself to show.
Where could be found to share our prince's state,
So fair, so virtuous, and so fit a mate?

See how the duckweed's stalks, or short or long,
Sway left and right, as moves the current strong!
So hard it was for him the maid to find!
By day, by night, our prince with constant mind
Sought for her long, but all his search was vain.
Awake, asleep, he ever felt the pain
Of longing thought, as when on restless bed,
Tossing about, one turns his fevered head.

Here long, there short, afloat the duckweed lies;
But caught at last, we seize the longed-for prize.
The maiden modest, virtuous, coy, is found;
Strike every lute, and joyous welcome sound.
Ours now, the duckweed from the stream we bear,
And cook to use with other viands rare.
He has the maiden, modest, virtuous, bright;
Let bells and drums proclaim our great delight

Celebrating the Industry of King Wan's Queen

Sweet was the scene. The spreading dolichos
Extended far, down to the valley's depths,
With leaves luxuriant. The orioles
Fluttered around, and on the bushy trees
In throngs collected—whence their pleasant notes
Resounded far in richest melody.

The spreading dolichos extended far,
Covering the valley's sides, down to its depths,
With leaves luxuriant and dense. I cut
It down, then boiled, and from the fibres spun
Of cloth, both fine and coarse, large store,
To wear, unwearied of such simple dress.

Now back to my old home, my parents dear
To see, I go. The matron I have told,
Who will announcement make. Meanwhile my clothes,
My private clothes I wash, and rinse my robes.
Which of them need be rinsed? and which need not?
My parents dear to visit, back I go.

In Praise of a Bride

Graceful and young the peach-tree stands;
  How rich its flowers, all gleaming bright!
This bride to her new home repairs;
  Chamber and house she'll order right.

Graceful and young the peach-tree stands;
  Large crops of fruit it soon will show.
This bride to her new home repairs;
  Chamber and house her sway shall know.

Graceful and young the peach-tree stands,
  Its foliage clustering green and full.
This bride to her new home repairs;
  Her household will attest her rule.

Celebrating T'ae-Sze's Freedom from Jealousy

In the South are the trees whose branches are bent,
And droop in such fashion that o'er their extent
  All the dolichos' creepers fast cling.
See our princely lady, from whom we have got
Rejoicing that's endless! May her happy lot
  And her honors repose ever bring!

In the South are the trees whose branches are bent,
And droop in such fashion that o'er their extent
  All the dolichos' creepers are spread.
See our princely lady, from whom we have got
Rejoicing that's endless! Of her happy lot
  And her honors the greatness ne'er fade!

In the South are the trees whose branches are bent,
And droop in such fashion that o'er their extent
  All the dolichos' creepers entwine.
See our princely lady, from whom we have got
Rejoicing that's endless! May her happy lot
  And her honors complete ever shine!

The Fruitfulness of the Locust

Ye locusts, winged tribes,
  Gather in concord fine;
Well your descendants may
  In numerous bright hosts shine!

Ye locusts, winged tribes,
  Your wings in flight resound;
Well your descendants may
  In endless lines be found!

Ye locusts, winged tribes,
  Together cluster strong;
Well your descendants may
  In swarms forever throng!

Lamenting the Absence of a Cherished Friend

Though small my basket, all my toil
  Filled it with mouse-ears but in part.
I set it on the path, and sighed
  For the dear master of my heart.

My steeds, o'er-tasked, their progress stayed,
  When midway up that rocky height.
Give me a cup from that gilt vase—
  When shall this longing end in sight?

To mount that lofty ridge I drove,
  Until my steeds all changed their hue.
A cup from that rhinoceros's horn
  May help my longing to subdue.

Striving to reach that flat-topped hill,
  My steeds, worn out, relaxed their strain;
My driver also sank oppressed:—
  I'll never see my lord again!

Celebrating the Goodness of the Descendants of King Wan

As the feet of the *lin*, which avoid each living thing,
So our prince's noble sons no harm to men will bring.
They are the *lin!*

As the front of the *lin*, never forward thrust in wrath,
So our prince's noble grandsons of love tread the path.
They are the *lin!*

As the horn of the *lin*, flesh-tipped, no wound to give,
So our prince's noble kindred kindly with all live.
They are the *lin!*

[NOTE.—The "lin" is the female of "K'e"—a fabulous animal—the symbol of all goodness and benevolence; having the body of a deer, the tail of an ox, the hoofs of a horse, one horn, the scales of a fish, *etc.* Its feet do not tread on any living thing—-not even on live grass; it does not butt with its forehead; and the end of its horn is covered with flesh—to show that, while able for war, it wills to have peace. The "lin" was supposed to appear inaugurating a golden age, but the poet finds a better auspice of that in the character of Wan's family and kindred.]

The Virtuous Manners of the Young Women

High and compressed, the Southern trees
 No shelter from the sun afford.
The girls free ramble by the Han,
 But will not hear enticing word.
Like the broad Han are they,
 Through which one cannot dive;
And like the Keang's long stream,
 Wherewith no raft can strive.

Many the fagots bound and piled;
 The thorns I'd hew still more to make.
As brides, those girls their new homes seek;
 Their colts to feed I'd undertake.
Like the broad Han are they,
 Through which one cannot dive;
And like the Keang's long stream,
 Wherewith no raft can strive.

Many the fagots bound and piled;
 The Southern-wood I'd cut for more.
As brides, those girls their new homes seek;
 Food for their colts I'd bring large store.
Like the broad Han are they,
 Through which one cannot dive;
And like the Keang's long stream,
 Wherewith no raft can strive.

Praise of a Rabbit-Catcher

Careful he sets his rabbit-nets all round;
Chang-chang his blows upon the pegs resound.
Stalwart the man and bold! his bearing all
Shows he might be his prince's shield and wall.

Careful he is his rabbit-nets to place
Where many paths of rabbits' feet bear trace.
Stalwart the man and bold! 'tis plain to see
He to his prince companion good would be.

Careful he is his rabbit-nets to spread,
Where in the forest's depth the trees give shade.
Stalwart the man and bold! fit his the part
Guide to his prince to be, and faithful heart.

The Song of the Plantain-Gatherers

We gather and gather the plantains;
  Come gather them anyhow.
Yes, gather and gather the plantains,
  And here we have got them now.

We gather and gather the plantains;
  Now off the ears we must tear.
Yes, gather and gather the plantains,
  And now the seeds are laid bare.

We gather and gather the plantains,
  The seeds in our skirts are placed.
Yes, gather and gather the plantains.
  Ho! safe in the girdled waist!

The Affection of the Wives on the Joo

Along the raised banks of the Joo,
  To hew slim stem and branch I wrought,
My lord away, my husband true,
  Like hunger-pang my troubled thought!

Along the raised banks of the Joo,
  Branch and fresh shoot confessed my art.
I've seen my lord, my husband true,
  And still he folds me in his heart.

As the toiled bream makes red its tail,
  Toil you, Sir, for the Royal House;

Amidst its blazing fires, nor quail:—
  Your parents see you pay your vows.

BOOK II

THE ODES OF SHAOU AND THE SOUTH

The Marriage of a Princess

  In the magpie's nest
  Dwells the dove at rest.
This young bride goes to her future home;
To meet her a hundred chariots come.

  Of the magpie's nest
  Is the dove possessed.
This bride goes to her new home to live;
And escort a hundred chariots give.

  The nest magpie wove
  Now filled by the dove.
This bride now takes to her home her way;
And these numerous cars her state display.

The Industry and Reverence of a Prince's Wife

Around the pools, the islets o'er,
  Fast she plucks white Southern-wood,
To help the sacrificial store;
  And for our prince does service good.

Where streams among the valleys shine,
  Of Southern-woods she plucks the white;
And brings it to the sacred shrine,
  To aid our prince in solemn rite.

In head-dress high, most reverent, she
  The temple seeks at early dawn.
The service o'er, the head-dress see
  To her own chamber slow withdrawn.

The Wife of Some Great Officer Bewails His Absence

Shrill chirp the insects in the grass;
  All about the hoppers spring.
While I my husband do not see,
  Sorrow must my bosom wring.
    O to meet him!

O to greet him!
Then my heart would rest and sing.

Ascending high that Southern hill,
Turtle ferns I strove to get.
While I my husband do not see,
Sorrow must my heart beset.
O to meet him!
O to greet him!
Then my heart would cease to fret.

Ascending high that Southern hill,
Spinous ferns I sought to find.
While I my husband do not see,
Rankles sorrow in my mind.
O to meet him!
O to greet him!
In my heart would peace be shrined.

The Diligence of the Young Wife of an Officer

She gathers fast the large duckweed,
From valley stream that southward flows;
And for the pondweed to the pools
Left on the plains by floods she goes.

The plants, when closed her toil, she puts
In baskets round and baskets square.
Then home she hies to cook her spoil,
In pans and tripods ready there.

In sacred chamber this she sets,
Where the light falls down through the wall.
'Tis she, our lord's young reverent wife,
Who manages this service all.

The Love of the People for the Duke of Shaou

O fell not that sweet pear-tree!
See how its branches spread.
Spoil not its shade,
For Shaou's chief laid
Beneath it his weary head.

O clip not that sweet pear-tree!
Each twig and leaflet spare.

'Tis sacred now,
Since the lord of Shaou,
When weary, rested him there.

O touch not that sweet pear-tree!
Bend not a twig of it now.
There long ago,
As the stories show,
Oft halted the chief of Shaou.

The Easy Dignity of the Officers at Some Court

Arrayed in skins of lamb or sheep,
With five silk braidings all of white,
From court they go, to take their meal,
All self-possessed, with spirits light.

How on their skins of lamb or sheep
The five seams wrought with white silk show!
With easy steps, and self-possessed,
From court to take their meal, they go.

Upon their skins of lamb or sheep
Shines the white silk the seams to link.
With easy steps and self-possessed,
They go from court to eat and drink.

Anxiety of a Young Lady to Get Married

Ripe, the plums fall from the bough;
Only seven-tenths left there now!
Ye whose hearts on me are set,
Now the time is fortunate!

Ripe, the plums fall from the bough;
Only three-tenths left there now!
Ye who wish my love to gain,
Will not now apply in vain!

No more plums upon the bough!
All are in my basket now!
Ye who me with ardor seek,
Need the word but freely speak!

BOOK III

THE ODES OF P'EI

An Officer Bewails the Neglect with which He is Treated

It floats about, that boat of cypress wood,
  Now here, now there, as by the current borne.
Nor rest nor sleep comes in my troubled mood;
  I suffer as when painful wound has torn
  The shrinking body. Thus I dwell forlorn,
And aimless muse, my thoughts of sorrow full.
  I might with wine refresh my spirit worn;
I might go forth, and, sauntering try to cool
The fever of my heart; but grief holds sullen rule.

My mind resembles not a mirror plate,
  Reflecting all the impressions it receives.
The good I love, the bad regard with hate;
  I only cherish whom my heart believes.
  Colleagues I have, but yet my spirit grieves,
That on their honor I cannot depend.
  I speak, but my complaint no influence leaves
Upon their hearts; with mine no feelings blend;
With me in anger they, and fierce disdain contend.

My mind is fixed, and cannot, like a stone,
  Be turned at will indifferently about;
And what I think, to that, and that alone,
  I utterance give, alike within, without;
  Nor can like mat be rolled and carried out.
With dignity in presence of them all,
  My conduct marked, my goodness who shall scout?
My foes I boldly challenge, great and small,
If there be aught in me they can in question call.

How full of trouble is my anxious heart!
  With hate the blatant herd of creatures mean
Ceaseless pursue. Of their attacks the smart
  Keeps my mind in distress. Their venomed spleen
  Aye vents itself; and with insulting mien
They vex my soul; and no one on my side
  A word will speak. Silent, alone, unseen,
I think of my sad case; then opening wide
My eyes, as if from sleep, I beat my breast, sore-tried.

Thy disc, O sun, should ever be complete,
  While thine, O changing moon, doth wax and wane.
But now our sun hath waned, weak and effete,
  And moons are ever full. My heart with pain
  Is firmly bound, and held in sorrow's chain,
As to the body cleaves an unwashed dress.
  Silent I think of my sad case; in vain
I try to find relief from my distress.
Would I had wings to fly where ills no longer press!

A Wife Deplores the Absence of Her Husband

Away the startled pheasant flies,
  With lazy movement of his wings.
Borne was my heart's lord from my eyes;—
  What pain the separation brings!

The pheasant, though no more in view,
  His cry, below, above, forth sends.
Alas! my princely lord, 'tis you—
  Your absence, that my bosom rends.

At sun and moon I sit and gaze,
  In converse with my troubled heart.
Far, far from me my husband stays!
  When will he come to heal its smart?

Ye princely men who with him mate,
  Say, mark ye not his virtuous way.
His rule is—covet nought, none hate;—
  How can his steps from goodness stray?

The Plaint of a Rejected Wife

The east wind gently blows,
  With cloudy skies and rain.
'Twixt man and wife should ne'er be strife,
  But harmony obtain.
Radish and mustard plants
  Are used, though some be poor;
While my good name is free from blame,
  Don't thrust me from your door.

I go along the road,
  Slow, with reluctant heart.
Your escort lame to door but came,

There glad from me to part.
Sow-thistle, bitter called,
As shepherd's purse is sweet;
With your new mate you feast elate,
As joyous brothers meet.

Part clear, the stream of King
Is foul beside the Wei.
You feast elate with your new mate,
And take no heed of me.
Loose mate, avoid my dam,
Nor dare my basket move!
Person slighted, life all blighted,
What can the future prove?

The water deep, in boat,
Or raft-sustained, I'd go;
And where the stream did narrow seem,
I dived or breasted through.
I labored to increase
Our means, or great or small;
When 'mong friends near death did appear,
On knees to help I'd crawl.

No cherishing you give,
I'm hostile in your eyes.
As pedler's wares for which none cares,
My virtues you despise.

When poverty was nigh,
I strove our means to spare;
You, now rich grown, me scorn to own;
To poison me compare.

The stores for winter piled
Are all unprized in spring.
So now, elate with your new mate,
Myself away you fling.
Your cool disdain for me
A bitter anguish hath.
The early time, our love's sweet prime,
In you wakes only wrath.

Soldiers of Wei Bewail Separation from Their Families

List to the thunder and roll of the drum!
See how we spring and brandish the dart!

Some raise Ts'aou's walls; some do field work at home;
But we to the southward lonely depart.

Our chief, Sun Tsze-chung, agreement has made,
Our forces to join with Ch'in and with Sung.
When shall we back from this service be led?
Our hearts are all sad, our courage unstrung.

Here we are halting, and there we delay;
Anon we soon lose our high-mettled steeds.
The forest's gloom makes our steps go astray;
Each thicket of trees our searching misleads.

For death as for life, at home or abroad,
We pledged to our wives our faithfulest word.
Their hands clasped in ours, together we vowed,
We'd live to old age in sweetest accord.

This march to the South can end but in ill;
Oh! never shall we our wives again meet.
The word that we pledged we cannot fulfil;
Us home returning they never will greet.

An Officer Tells of His Mean Employment

With mind indifferent, things I easy take;
In every dance I prompt appearance make:—
Then, when the sun is at his topmost height,
There, in the place that courts the public sight.

With figure large I in the courtyard dance,
And the duke smiles, when he beholds me prance.
A tiger's strength I have; the steeds swift bound;
The reins as ribbons in my hands are found.

See how I hold the flute in my left hand;
In right the pheasant's plume, waved like a wand;
With visage red, where rouge you think to trace,
While the duke pleased, sends down the cup of grace!

Hazel on hills; the *ling* in meadow damp;—
Each has its place, while I'm a slighted scamp.
My thoughts go back to th' early days of Chow,
And muse upon its chiefs, not equalled now.
O noble chiefs, who then the West adorned,
Would ye have thus neglected me and scorned?

An Officer Sets Forth His Hard Lot

My way leads forth by the gate on the north;
 My heart is full of woe.
I hav'n't a cent, begged, stolen, or lent,
 And friends forget me so.
  So let it be! 'tis Heaven's decree.
  What can I say—a poor fellow like me?

The King has his throne, sans sorrow or moan;
 On me fall all his cares,
And when I come home, resolved not to roam,
 Each one indignant stares.
  So let it be! 'tis Heaven's decree.
  What can I say—a poor fellow like me?

Each thing of the King, and the fate of the State,
 On me come more and more.
And when, sad and worn, I come back forlorn,
 They thrust me from the door.
  So let it be! 'tis Heaven's decree.
  What can I say—a poor fellow like me?

The Complaint of a Neglected Wife

When the upper robe is green,
With a yellow lining seen,
There we have a certain token,
Right is wronged and order broken.
How can sorrow from my heart
In a case like this depart?

Color green the robe displays;
Lower garment yellow's blaze.
Thus it is that favorite mean
In the place of wife is seen.
Vain the conflict with my grief;
Memory denies relief.

Yes, 'twas you the green who dyed,
You who fed the favorite's pride.
Anger rises in my heart,
Pierces it as with a dart.
But on ancient rules lean I,
Lest to wrong my thoughts should fly.

Fine or coarse, if thin the dress,
Cold winds always cause distress.
Hard my lot, my sorrow deep,
But my thoughts in check I keep.
Ancient story brings to mind
Sufferers who were resigned.

[NOTE.—Yellow is one of the five "correct" colors of the Chinese, while green is one of the "intermediate" colors that are less esteemed. Here we have the yellow used merely as a lining to the green, or employed in the lower, or less honorable, part of the dress;—an inversion of propriety, and intimating how a favorite had usurped the place of the rightful wife and thrust her down.]

In Praise of a Maiden

O sweet maiden, so fair and retiring,
  At the corner I'm waiting for you;
And I'm scratching my head, and inquiring
  What on earth it were best I should do.

Oh! the maiden, so handsome and coy,
  For a pledge gave a slim rosy reed.
Than the reed is she brighter, my joy;
  On her loveliness how my thoughts feed!

In the pastures a *t'e* blade she sought,
  And she gave it, so elegant, rare.
Oh! the grass does not dwell in my thought,
  But the donor, more elegant, fair.

Discontent

As when the north winds keenly blow,
And all around fast falls the snow,
The source of pain and suffering great,
So now it is in Wei's poor state.
Let us join hands and haste away,
  My friends and lovers all.
'Tis not a time will brook delay;
  Things for prompt action call.

As when the north winds whistle shrill,
And drifting snows each hollow fill,
The source of pain and suffering great,
So now it is in Wei's poor state,
Let us join hands, and leave for aye,

My friends and lovers all,
'Tis not a time will brook delay;
Things for prompt action call.

We look for red, and foxes meet;
For black, and crows our vision greet.
The creatures, both of omen bad,
Well suit the state of Wei so sad.

Let us join hands and mount our cars,
My friends and lovers all.
No time remains for wordy jars;
Things for prompt action call.

Chwang Keang Bemoans Her Husband's Cruelty

Fierce is the wind and cold;
And such is he.
Smiling he looks, and bold
Speaks mockingly.
Scornful and lewd his words,
Haughty his smile.
Bound is my heart with cords
In sorrow's coil.

As cloud of dust wind-blown,
Just such is he.
Ready he seems to own,
And come to me.
But he comes not nor goes,
Stands in his pride.
Long, long, with painful throes,
Grieved I abide.

Strong blew the wind; the cloud
Hastened away.
Soon dark again, the shroud
Covers the day.
I wake, and sleep no more
Visits my eyes.
His course I sad deplore,
With heavy sighs.

Cloudy the sky, and dark;
The thunders roll.
Such outward signs well mark
My troubled soul.

I wake, and sleep no more
  Comes to give rest.
His course I sad deplore,
  In anguished breast.

[NOTE: Selections from Books IV., V., and VI., have been omitted.—EDITOR.]

BOOK VII

THE ODES OF CH'ING

The People's Admiration for Duke Woo

The black robes well your form befit;
  When they are worn we'll make you new.
Now for your court! oh! there we'll sit,
  And watch how you your duties do.
    And when we to our homes repair,
    We'll send to you our richest fare,
    Such is the love to you we bear!

Those robes well with your virtue match;
  When they are worn we'll make you new.
Now for your court! There will we watch,
  Well pleased, how you your duties do.
    And when we to our homes repair,
    We'll send to you our richest fare,
    Such is the love to you we bear!

Those robes your character beseem;
  When they are worn we'll make you new.
Now for your court! oh! there we deem
  It pleasure great your form to view.
    And when we to our homes repair,
    We'll send to you our richest fare,
    Such is the love to you we bear!

A Wife Consoled by Her Husband's Arrival

Cold is the wind, fast falls the rain,
  The cock aye shrilly crows.
But I have seen my lord again;—
  Now must my heart repose.

Whistles the wind, patters the rain,
  The cock's crow far resounds.
But I have seen my lord again,
  And healed are my heart's wounds.

All's dark amid the wind and rain,
  Ceaseless the cock's clear voice!
But I have seen my lord again;—
  Should not my heart rejoice?

In Praise of Some Lady

There by his side in chariot rideth she,
As lovely flower of the hibiscus tree,
So fair her face; and when about they wheel,
Her girdle gems of *Ken* themselves reveal.
For beauty all the House of Keang have fame;
Its eldest daughter—she beseems her name.

There on the path, close by him, walketh she,
Bright as the blossom of hibiscus tree,
And fair her face; and when around they flit,
Her girdle gems a tinkling sound emit.
Among the Keang she has distinguished place,
For virtuous fame renowned, and peerless grace.

A Man's Praise of His Wife

My path forth from the east gate lay,
Where cloud-like moved the girls at play.
Numerous are they, as clouds so bright,
But not on them my heart's thoughts light.
Dressed in a thin white silk, with coiffure gray
Is she, my wife, my joy in life's low way.

Forth by the covering wall's high tower,
I went, and saw, like rush in flower,
Each flaunting girl. Brilliant are they,
But not with them my heart's thoughts stay.
In thin white silk, with head-dress madder-dyed,
Is she, my sole delight, 'foretime my bride.

An Entreaty

Along the great highway,
 I hold you by the cuff.
O spurn me not, I pray,
 Nor break old friendship off.

Along the highway worn,
 I hold your hand in mine.
Do not as vile me scorn;
 Your love I can't resign.

A Woman Scorning Her Lover

O dear! that artful boy
 Refuses me a word!
But, Sir, I shall enjoy
 My food, though you're absurd!

O dear! that artful boy
 My table will not share!
But, Sir, I shall enjoy
 My rest, though you're not there!

A Lady Mourns the Absence of Her Student Lover

You student, with the collar blue,
 Long pines my heart with anxious pain.
Although I do not go to you,
 Why from all word do you refrain?

O you, with girdle strings of blue,
 My thoughts to you forever roam!
Although I do not go to you,
 Yet why to me should you not come?

How reckless you, how light and wild,
 There by the tower upon the wall!
One day, from sight of you exiled,
 As long as three long months I call.

[NOTE: Selections from Books IV., V., and VI., have been omitted.—EDITOR.]

BOOK VIII

THE ODES OF TS'E

A Wife Urging Her Husband to Action

His lady to the marquis says,
  "The cock has crowed; 'tis late.
Get up, my lord, and haste to court.
  'Tis full; for you they wait."
She did not hear the cock's shrill sound,
Only the blueflies buzzing round.

Again she wakes him with the words,
  "The east, my lord, is bright.
A crowded court your presence seeks;
  Get up and hail the light."
'Twas not the dawning light which shone,
But that which by the moon was thrown.

He sleeping still, once more she says,
  "The flies are buzzing loud.
To lie and dream here by your side
  Were pleasant, but the crowd
Of officers will soon retire;
Draw not on you and me their ire!"

The Folly of Useless Effort

The weeds will but the ranker grow,
  If fields too large you seek to till.
To try to gain men far away
  With grief your toiling heart will fill,

If fields too large you seek to till,
  The weeds will only rise more strong.
To try to gain men far away
  Will but your heart's distress prolong.

Things grow the best when to themselves
  Left, and to nature's vigor rare.
How young and tender is the child,
  With his twin tufts of falling hair!
But when you him ere long behold,
  That child shall cap of manhood wear!

The Prince of Loo

A grand man is the prince of Loo,
 With person large and high.
Lofty his front and suited to
 The fine glance of his eye!
Swift are his feet. In archery
 What man with him can vie?
With all these goodly qualities,
 We see him and we sigh!

Renowned through all the land is he,
 The nephew of our lord.
With clear and lovely eyes, his grace
 May not be told by word.
All day at target practice,
 He'll never miss the bird.
Such is the prince of Loo, and yet
 With grief for him we're stirred!

All grace and beauty he displays,
 High forehead and eyes bright.
And dancing choice! His arrows all
 The target hit aright.
Straight through they go, and every one
 Lights on the self-same spot.
Rebellion he could well withstand,
 And yet we mourn his lot!

BOOK IX

THE ODES OF WEI

On the Misgovernment of the State

A fruit, small as the garden peach,
  May still be used for food.
A State, though poor as ours, might thrive,
  If but its rule were good.
Our rule is bad, our State is sad,
  With mournful heart I grieve.
All can from instrument and voice
  My mood of mind perceive.
Who know me not, with scornful thought,
  Deem me a scholar proud.
"Those men are right," they fiercely say,
  "What mean your words so loud?"
Deep in my heart my sorrows lie,
  And none the cause may know.
How should they know who never try
  To learn whence comes our woe?

The garden jujube, although small,
  May still be used for food.
A State, though poor as ours, might thrive,
  If but its rule were good.
Our rule is bad, our State is sad,
  With mournful heart I grieve.
Methinks I'll wander through the land,
  My misery to relieve.
Who know me not, with scornful thought,
  Deem that wild views I hold.
"Those men are right," they fiercely say,
  "What mean your words so bold?"

Deep in my heart my sorrows lie,
And none the cause may know.
How can they know, who never try
To learn whence comes our woe?

The Mean Husband

Thin cloth of dolichos supplies the shoes,
  In which some have to brave the frost and cold.
A bride, when poor, her tender hands must use,

Her dress to make, and the sharp needle hold.
This man is wealthy, yet he makes his bride
Collars and waistbands for his robes provide.

Conscious of wealth, he moves with easy mien;
Politely on the left he takes his place;
The ivory pin is at his girdle seen:—
His dress and gait show gentlemanly grace.
Why do we brand him in our satire here?
'Tis this—his niggard soul provokes the sneer.

A Young Soldier on Service

To the top of that tree-clad hill I go,
And towards my father I gaze,
Till with my mind's eye his form I espy,
And my mind's ear hears how he says:—
"Alas for my son on service abroad!
He rests not from morning till eve.
May he careful be and come back to me!
While he is away, how I grieve!"

To the top of that barren hill I climb,
And towards my mother I gaze,
Till with my mind's eye her form I espy,
And my mind's ear hears how she says:—
"Alas for my child on service abroad!
He never in sleep shuts an eye.
May he careful be, and come back to me!
In the wild may his body not lie!"

Up the lofty ridge I, toiling, ascend,
And towards my brother I gaze,
Till with my mind's eye his form I espy,
And my mind's ear hears how he says:—
"Alas! my young brother, serving abroad,
All day with his comrades must roam.
May he careful be, and come back to me,
And die not away from his home."

BOOK X

THE ODES OF TANG

The King Goes to War

The wild geese fly the bushy oaks around,
With clamor loud. *Suh-suh* their wings resound,
As for their feet poor resting-place is found.
The King's affairs admit of no delay.
Our millet still unsown, we haste away.
No food is left our parents to supply;
When we are gone, on whom can they rely?
O azure Heaven, that shinest there afar,
When shall our homes receive us from the war?

The wild geese on the bushy jujube-trees Attempt to settle and are ill at ease;— *Suh-suh* their wings go flapping in the breeze. The King's affairs admit of no delay; Our millet still unsown, we haste away. How shall our parents their requirements get? How in our absence shall their wants be met? O azure Heaven, that shinest there afar, When shall our homes receive us from the war?

The bushy mulberry-trees the geese in rows
Seek eager and to rest around them close—
With rustling loud, as disappointment grows.
The King's affairs admit of no delay;
To plant our rice and maize we cannot stay.
How shall our parents find their wonted food?
When we are gone, who will to them be good?
O azure Heaven, that shinest there afar,
When shall our homes receive us from the war?

Lament of a Bereaved Person

A russet pear-tree rises all alone,
But rich the growth of leaves upon it shown!
I walk alone, without one brother left,
And thus of natural aid am I bereft.
Plenty of people there are all around,
But none like my own father's sons are found.
Ye travellers, who forever hurry by,
Why on me turn the unsympathizing eye?

No brother lives with whom my cause to plead;—
Why not perform for me the helping deed?

A russet pear-tree rises all alone,
But rich with verdant foliage o'ergrown.
I walk alone, without one brother's care,
To whom I might, amid my straits repair.
Plenty of people there are all around,
But none like those of my own name are found.
Ye travellers, who forever hurry by,
Why on me turn the unsympathizing eye?
No brother lives with whom my cause to plead;—
Why not perform for me the helping deed?

The Drawbacks of Poverty

On the left of the way, a russet pear-tree
Stands there all alone—a fit image of me.
There is that princely man! O that he would come,
And in my poor dwelling with me be at home!
In the core of my heart do I love him, but say,
Whence shall I procure him the wants of the day?

At the bend in the way a russet pear-tree
Stands there all alone—a fit image of me.
There is that princely man! O that he would come,
And rambling with me be himself here at home!
In the core of my heart I love him, but say,
Whence shall I procure him the wants of the day?

A Wife Mourns for Her Husband

The dolichos grows and covers the thorn,
  O'er the waste is the dragon-plant creeping.
The man of my heart is away and I mourn—
  What home have I, lonely and weeping?

Covering the jujubes the dolichos grows,
  The graves many dragon-plants cover;
But where is the man on whose breast I'd repose?
  No home have I, having no lover!

Fair to see was the pillow of horn,
  And fair the bed-chamber's adorning;
But the man of my heart is not here, and I mourn
  All alone, and wait for the morning.

While the long days of summer pass over my head,
  And long winter nights leave their traces,
I'm alone! Till a hundred of years shall have fled,
  And then I shall meet his embraces.

Through the long winter nights I am burdened with fears,
  Through the long summer days I am lonely;
But when time shall have counted its hundreds of years
  I then shall be his—and his only!

BOOK XI

THE ODES OF TS'IN

Celebrating the Opulence of the Lords of Ts'in

Our ruler to the hunt proceeds;
And black as iron are his steeds
That heed the charioteer's command,
Who holds the six reins in his hand.
His favorites follow to the chase,
Rejoicing in his special grace.

The season's males, alarmed, arise—
The season's males, of wondrous size.
Driven by the beaters, forth they spring,
Soon caught within the hunters' ring.
"Drive on their left," the ruler cries;
And to its mark his arrow flies.

The hunting done, northward he goes;
And in the park the driver shows
The horses' points, and his own skill
That rules and guides them at his will.
Light cars whose teams small bells display,
The long-and short-mouthed dogs convey.

A Complaint

He lodged us in a spacious house,
  And plenteous was our fare.
But now at every frugal meal
  There's not a scrap to spare.
Alas! alas that this good man
Could not go on as he began!

A Wife's Grief Because of Her Husband's Absence

The falcon swiftly seeks the north,
And forest gloom that sent it forth.
Since I no more my husband see,
My heart from grief is never free.
O how is it, I long to know,
That he, my lord, forgets me so?

Bushy oaks on the mountain grow,
And six elms where the ground is low.
But I, my husband seen no more,
My sad and joyless fate deplore.
O how is it, I long to know,
That he, my lord, forgets me so?

The hills the bushy wild plums show,
And pear-trees grace the ground below.
But, with my husband from me gone,
As drunk with grief, I dwell alone.
O how is it, I long to know,
That he, my lord, forgets me so?

Lament for Three Brothers

They flit about, the yellow birds,
  And rest upon the jujubes find.
Who buried were in duke Muh's grave,
  Alive to awful death consigned?

'Mong brothers three, who met that fate,
  'Twas sad the first, Yen-seih to see.
He stood alone; a hundred men
  Could show no other such as he.
When to the yawning grave he came,
Terror unnerved and shook his frame.

Why thus destroy our noblest men,
  To thee we cry, O azure Heaven!
To save Yen-seih from death, we would
  A hundred lives have freely given.

They flit about, the yellow birds,
  And on the mulberry-trees rest find.
Who buried were in duke Muh's grave,
  Alive to awful death consigned?

'Mong brothers three, who met that fate,
  'Twas sad the next, Chung-hang to see.
When on him pressed a hundred men,
  A match for all of them was he.
When to the yawning grave he came,
Terror unnerved and shook his frame.

Why thus destroy our noblest men,
 To thee we cry, O azure Heaven!
To save Chung-hang from death, we would
 A hundred lives have freely given.

They flit about, the yellow birds,
 And rest upon the thorn-trees find.
Who buried were in duke Muh's grave,
 Alive to awful death consigned?

'Mong brothers three, who met that fate,
 'Twas sad the third, K'een-foo, to see.
A hundred men in desperate fight
 Successfully withstand could he.
When to the yawning grave he came,
Terror unnerved and shook his frame.

Why thus destroy our noblest men,
 To thee we cry, O azure Heaven!
To save K'een-foo from death, we would
 A hundred lives have freely given.

[NOTE.—The incident related in this poem occurred in the year B.C. 620, when the duke of Muh died after playing an important part in the affairs of Northwest China. Muh required the three officers here celebrated, to be buried with him, and according to the "Historical Records" this barbarous practice began with duke Ching, Muh's predecessor. In all, 170 individuals were buried with Muh. The death of the last distinguished man of the Ts'in dynasty, the Emperor I, was subsequently celebrated by the entombment with him of all the inmates of his harem.]

In Praise of a Ruler of Ts'in

What trees grow on the Chung-nan hill?
 The white fir and the plum.
In fur of fox, 'neath 'broidered robe,
 Thither our prince is come.
His face glows with vermilion hue.
O may he prove a ruler true!

What find we on the Chung-nan hill?
 Deep nook and open glade.
Our prince shows there the double *Ke*
 On lower robe displayed.
His pendant holds each tinkling gem,
Long life be his, and deathless fame!

The Generous Nephew

I escorted my uncle to Tsin,
  Till the Wei we crossed on the way.
    Then I gave as I left
    For his carriage a gift
Four steeds, and each steed was a bay.

I escorted my uncle to Tsin,
  And I thought of him much in my heart.
    Pendent stones, and with them
   Of fine jasper a gem,
I gave, and then saw him depart.

BOOK XII

THE ODES OF CH'IN

The Contentment of a Poor Recluse

My only door some pieces of crossed wood,
 Within it I can rest enjoy.
I drink the water wimpling from the spring;
 Nor hunger can my peace destroy.

Purged from ambition's aims I say, "For fish.
 We need not bream caught in the Ho;
Nor, to possess the sweets of love, require
 To Ts'e, to find a Keang, to go.

"The man contented with his lot, a meal
 Of fish without Ho carp can make;
Nor needs, to rest in his domestic joy,
 A Tsze of Sung as wife to take."

The Disappointed Lover

Where grow the willows near the eastern gate,
 And 'neath their leafy shade we could recline,
She said at evening she would me await,
 And brightly now I see the day-star shine!

Here where the willows near the eastern gate
 Grow, and their dense leaves make a shady gloom,
She said at evening she would me await.
 See now the morning star the sky illume!

A Love-Song

The moon comes forth, bright in the sky;
A lovelier sight to draw my eye
 Is she, that lady fair.
She round my heart has fixed love's chain,
But all my longings are in vain.
 'Tis hard the grief to bear.

The moon comes forth, a splendid sight;
More winning far that lady bright,
 Object of my desire!

Deep-seated is my anxious grief;
In vain I seek to find relief;
  While glows the secret fire.

The rising moon shines mild and fair;
More bright is she, whose beauty rare
  My heart with longing fills.
With eager wish I pine in vain;
O for relief from constant pain,
  Which through my bosom thrills!

The Lament of a Lover

There where its shores the marsh surround,
Rushes and lotus plants abound.
Their loveliness brings to my mind
The lovelier one that I would find.
In vain I try to ease the smart
Of wounded love that wrings my heart.
In waking thought and nightly dreams,
From every pore the water streams.

All round the marsh's shores are seen
Valerian flowers and rushes green.
But lovelier is that Beauty rare,
Handsome and large, and tall and fair,
I wish and long to call her mine,
Doomed with the longing still to pine.
Nor day nor night e'er brings relief;
My inmost heart is full of grief.

Around the marsh, in rich display,
Grow rush and lotus flowers, all gay.
But not with her do they compare,
So tall and large, majestic, fair.
Both day and night, I nothing speed;
Still clings to me the aching need.
On side, on back, on face, I lie,
But vain each change of posture.

THE ODES OF KWEI

The Wish of an Unhappy Man

Where the grounds are wet and low,
There the trees of goat-peach grow,
With their branches small and smooth,
Glossy in their tender youth.
Joy it were to me, O tree,
Consciousness to want like thee.

Where the grounds are wet and low,
There the trees of goat-peach grow.
Soft and fragrant are their flowers,
Glossy from the vernal showers.
Joy it were to me, O tree,
Ties of home to want like thee.

Where the grounds are wet and low,
There the trees of goat-peach grow,
What delicious fruits they bear,
Glossy, soft, of beauty rare!
Joy it were to me, O tree,
Household cares to want like thee.

BOOK XIV

THE ODES OF TS'AOU

Against Frivolous Pursuits

Like splendid robes appear the wings
  Of the ephemeral fly;
And such the pomp of those great men,
  Which soon in death shall lie!
I grieve! Would they but come to me!
  To teach them I should try.

The wings of the ephemeral fly
  Are robes of colors gay;
And such the glory of those men,
  Soon crumbling to decay!
I grieve! Would they but rest with me,
  They'd learn a better way!

The ephemeral fly bursts from its hole,
  With gauzy wings like snow;
So quick the rise, so quick the fall,
  Of those great men we know!
I grieve! Would they but lodge with me,
  Forth they would wiser go.

BOOK XV

THE ODES OF PIN

The Duke of Chow Tells of His Soldiers

To the hills of the east we went,
  And long had we there to remain.
When the word of recall was sent,
  Thick and fast came the drizzling rain.
When told our return we should take,
  Our hearts in the West were and sore;
But there did they clothes for us make:—
  They knew our hard service was o'er.
On the mulberry grounds in our sight
  The large caterpillars were creeping;
Lonely and still we passed the night,
  All under our carriages sleeping.

To the hills of the East we went,
  And long had we there to remain.
When the word of recall was sent,
  Thick and fast came the drizzling rain.
The heavenly gourds rise to the eye,
  With their fruit hanging under the eave.
In our chambers the sow-bug we spy;
  Their webs on our doors spiders weave.
Our paddocks seem crowded with deer,
  With the glow-worm's light all about.
Such thoughts, while they filled us with fear,
  We tried, but in vain, to keep out.

To the hills of the East we went,
  And long had we there to remain.
When the word of recall was sent,
  Thick and fast came the drizzling rain.

On ant-hills screamed cranes with delight;
  In their rooms were our wives sighing sore.
Our homes they had swept and made tight:—
  All at once we arrived at the door.
The bitter gourds hanging are seen,
  From branches of chestnut-trees high.
Three years of toil away we had been,
  Since such a sight greeted the eye.

To the hills of the East we went,
 And long had we there to remain.
When the word of recall was sent,
 Thick and fast came the drizzling rain.
With its wings now here, and now there,
 Is the oriole sporting in flight.
Those brides to their husbands repair,
 Their steeds red and bay, flecked with white.
Each mother has fitted each sash;
 Their equipments are full and complete;
But fresh unions, whatever their dash,
 Can ne'er with reunions compete.

There is a Proper Way for Doing Everything

In hewing an axe-shaft, how must you act?
 Another axe take, or you'll never succeed.
In taking a wife, be sure 'tis a fact,
 That with no go-between you never can speed.

In hewing an axe-shaft, hewing a shaft,
 For a copy you have the axe in your hand.

In choosing a wife, you follow the craft,
 And forthwith on the mats the feast-vessels stand.

PART II.—MINOR ODES TO THE KINGDOM

BOOK I

DECADE OF LUH MING

A Festal Ode

With sounds of happiness the deer
  Browse on the celery of the meads.
A nobler feast is furnished here,
  With guests renowned for noble deeds.
The lutes are struck; the organ blows,
  Till all its tongues in movement heave.
Each basket loaded stands, and shows
  The precious gifts the guests receive.
They love me and my mind will teach,
How duty's highest aim to reach.

With sounds of happiness the deer
  The southern-wood crop in the meads,
What noble guests surround me here,
  Distinguished for their worthy deeds!
From them my people learn to fly
  Whate'er is mean; to chiefs they give
A model and a pattern high;—
  They show the life they ought to live.
Then fill their cups with spirits rare,
Till each the banquet's joy shall share.

With sounds of happiness the deer
  The salsola crop in the fields.
What noble guests surround me here!
  Each lute for them its music yields.
Sound, sound the lutes, or great or small.
  The joy harmonious to prolong;—

And with my spirits rich crown all
  The cups to cheer the festive throng.
Let each retire with gladdened heart,
In his own sphere to play his part.

A Festal Ode Complimenting an Officer

On dashed my four steeds, without halt, without stay,
Though toilsome and winding from Chow was the way.
I wished to return—but the monarch's command

Forbade that his business be done with slack hand;
  And my heart was with sadness oppressed.

On dashed my four steeds; I ne'er slackened the reins.
They snorted and panted—all white, with black manes.
I wished to return, but our sovereign's command
Forbade that his business be done with slack hand;—
  And I dared not to pause or to rest.

Unresting the Filial doves speed in their flight,
Ascending, then sweeping swift down from the height,
Now grouped on the oaks. The king's high command
Forbade that his business be done with slack hand;—
  And my father I left, sore distressed.

Unresting the Filial doves speed in their flight,
Now fanning the air and anon they alight
On the medlars thick grouped. But our monarch's command
Forbade that his business be done with slack hand;—
  Of my mother I thought with sad breast.

My four steeds I harnessed, all white and black-maned,
Which straight on their way, fleet and emulous strained.
I wished to return; and now venture in song
The wish to express, and announce how I long
  For my mother my care to attest.

[NOTE.—Both Maou and Choo agree that this ode was composed in honor of the officer who narrates the story in it, although they say it was not written by the officer himself, but was put into his mouth, as it were, to express the sympathy of his entertainer with him, and the appreciation of his devotion to duty.]

The Value of Friendship

The woodmen's blows responsive ring,
  As on the trees they fall;
And when the birds their sweet notes sing,
  They to each other call.
From the dark valley comes a bird,
  And seeks the lofty tree.
Ying goes its voice, and thus it cries,
  "Companion, come to me."
The bird, although a creature small,
  Upon its mate depends;
And shall we men, who rank o'er all,
  Not seek to have our friends?
All spirits love the friendly man,

And hearken to his prayer.
What harmony and peace they can
Bestow, his lot shall share.

Hoo-hoo the woodmen all unite
To shout, as trees they fell.
They do their work with all their might;—
What I have done I'll tell.
I've strained and made my spirits clear,
The fatted lambs I've killed.
With friends who my own surname bear,
My hall I've largely filled.
Some may be absent, casually,
And leave a broken line;
But better this than absence by
An oversight of mine.
My court I've sprinkled and swept clean,
Viands in order set.
Eight dishes loaded stand with grain;
There's store of fatted meat.
My mother's kith and kin I'm sure
I've widely called by name.
That some be hindered better is
Than *I* give cause for blame.

On the hill-side the trees they fell,
All working with good-will
I labor too, with equal zeal.
And the host's part fulfil.
Spirits I've set in order meet,
The dishes stand in rows.
The guests are here; no vacant seat
A brother absent shows.
The loss of kindly feeling oft
From slightest things shall grow,
Where all the fare is dry and spare,
Resentments fierce may glow.
My store of spirits is well strained,
If short prove the supply,
My messengers I straightway send,
And what is needed buy.
I beat the drums, and in the dance
Lead joyously the train.
Oh! good it is, when falls the chance
The sparkling cup to drain.

The Response to a Festal Ode

Heaven shields and sets thee fast.
It round thee fair has cast
  Thy virtue pure.
Thus richest joy is thine;—
Increase of corn and wine,
And every gift divine,
  Abundant, sure.

Heaven shields and sets thee fast.
From it thou goodness hast;
  Right are thy ways.
Its choicest gifts 'twill pour,
That last for evermore,
Nor time exhaust the store
  Through endless days.

Heaven shields and sets thee fast,
Makes thine endeavor last
  And prosper well.
Like hills and mountains high,
Whose masses touch the sky;
Like streams aye surging by;
  Thine increase swell!

With rite and auspice fair,
Thine offerings thou dost bear,
  And son-like give,
The season's round from spring,
To olden duke and king,
Whose words to thee we bring:—
  "Forever live,"

The spirits of thy dead
Pour blessings on thy head,
  Unnumbered sweet.
Thy subjects, simple, good,
Enjoy their drink and food.
Our tribes of every blood
  Follow thy feet.

Like moons that wax in light;
Or suns that scale the height;
  Or ageless hill;
Nor change, nor autumn know;
As pine and cypress grow;
The sons that from thee flow
  Be lasting still!

An Ode of Congratulation

The russet pear-tree stands there all alone;
How bright the growth of fruit upon it shown!
The King's affairs no stinting hands require,
And days prolonged still mock our fond desire.
But time has brought the tenth month of the year;
My woman's heart is torn with wound severe.
Surely my warrior lord might now appear!

The russet pear-tree stands there all alone;
How dense the leafy shade all o'er it thrown!
The King's affairs require no slackening hand,
And our sad hearts their feelings can't command.
The plants and trees in beauty shine; 'tis spring.
From off my heart its gloom I fain would fling.
This season well my warrior home may bring!

I climbed that northern hill, and medlars sought;
The spring nigh o'er, to ripeness they were brought.
"The King's affairs cannot be slackly done";—
'Tis thus our parents mourn their absent son.
But now his sandal car must broken be;
I seem his powerful steeds worn out to see.
Relief has gone! He can't be far from me!

Alas! they can't have marched; they don't arrive!
More hard it grows with my distress to strive.
The time is passed, and still he is not here!
My sorrows multiply; great is my fear.
But lo! by reeds and shell I have divined,
That he is near, they both assure my mind;—
Soon at my side my warrior I shall find!

An Ode on the Return of the Troops

Forth from the city in our cars we drove,
  Until we halted at the pasture ground.
The general came, and there with ardor strove
  A note of zeal throughout the host to sound.
  "Direct from court I come, by orders bound
The march to hasten";—it was thus he spake.
  Then with the carriage-officers around,
He strictly charged them quick despatch to make:—
"Urgent the King's affairs, forthwith the field we take."

While there we stopped, the second corps appeared,
And 'twixt Us and the city took its place.
The guiding standard was on high upreared,
Where twining snakes the tortoises embrace,
While oxtails, crest-like, did the staff's top grace.
We watched the sheet unfolding grandly wave;
Each flag around showed falcons on its face.

With anxious care looked on our leader brave;
Watchful the carriage-officers appeared and grave.

Nan Chung, our chief, had heard the royal call
To go where inroad by Heen-yuns was made,
And 'cross the frontier build a barrier wall.
Numerous his chariots, splendidly arrayed!
The standards—this where dragons were displayed,
And that where snakes round tortoises were coiled—
Terrific flew. "Northward our host," he said,
"Heaven's son sends forth to tame the Heen-yun wild."
Soon by this awful chief would all their tribes be foiled.

When first we took the field, and northward went,
The millet was in flower;—a prospect sweet.
Now when our weary steps are homeward bent,
The snow falls fast, the mire impedes our feet.
Many the hardships we were called to meet,
Ere the King's orders we had all fulfilled.
No rest we had; often our friends to greet
The longing came; but vain regrets we stilled;
By tablets stern our hearts with fresh resolve were thrilled.

"Incessant chirp the insects in the grass;
All round about the nimble hoppers spring.
From them our thoughts quick to our husbands pass?
Although those thoughts our hearts with anguish wring.
Oh! could we see them, what relief 'twould bring!
Our hearts, rejoiced, at once would feel at rest."
Thus did our wives, their case deploring, sing;
The while our leader farther on had pressed,
And smitten with his power the wild Jung of the west.

The spring days now are lengthening out their light;
The plants and trees are dressed in living green;
The orioles resting sing, or wing their flight;
Our wives amid the southern-wood are seen,
Which white they bring, to feed their silkworms keen.
Our host, returned, sweeps onwards to the hall,

Where chiefs are questioned, shown the captives mean
Nan Chung, majestic, draws the gaze of all,
Proud o'er the barbarous foe his victories to recall.

BOOK II

THE DECADE OF PIH H'WA

An Ode Appropriate to a Festivity

The dew lies heavy all around,
Nor, till the sun shines, leaves the ground.
Far into night we feasting sit;
We drink, and none his place may quit.

The dew lies heavy, and its gems
Stud the luxuriant, grassy stems.
The happy night with wassail rings;
So feasted here the former kings.

The jujube and the willow-tree
All fretted with the dew we see.
Each guest's a prince of noble line,
In whom the virtues all combine.

The *t'ung* and *e* their fruits display,
Pendant from every graceful spray.
My guests are joyous and serene,
No haggard eye, no ruffled mien.

BOOK III

THE DECADE OF TUNG RUNG

Celebrating a Hunting Expedition

Our chariots were well-built and firm,
Well-matched our steeds, and fleet and strong.
Four, sleek and large, each chariot drew,
And eastward thus we drove along.

Our hunting cars were light and good,
Each with its team of noble steeds.
Still further east we took the way
To Foo-mere's grassy plains that leads.

Loud-voiced, the masters of the chase
Arranged the huntsmen, high and low.
While banners streamed, and ox-tails flew,
We sought the prey on distant Gaou.

Each with full team, the princes came,
A lengthened train in bright array.
In gold-wrought slippers, knee-caps red,
They looked as on an audience day.

Each right thumb wore the metal guard;
On the left arm its shield was bound.
In unison the arrows flew;
The game lay piled upon the ground.

The leaders of the tawny teams
Sped on their course, direct and true.
The drivers perfect skill displayed;
Like blow well aimed each arrow flew.

Neighing and pleased, the steeds returned;
The bannered lines back slowly came.
No jostling rude disgraced the crowd;
The king declined large share of game.

So did this famous hunt proceed!
So free it was from clamorous sound!
Well does our King become his place,
And high the deeds his reign have crowned!

The King's Anxiety for His Morning Levee

How goes the night? For heavy morning sleep
Ill suits the king who men would loyal keep.
The courtyard, ruddy with the torch's light,
Proclaims unspent the deepest hour of night.
Already near the gate my lords appear;
Their tinkling bells salute my wakeful ear.

How goes the night? I may not slumber on.
Although not yet the night is wholly gone,
The paling torch-light in the court below
Gives token that the hours swift-footed go.
Already at the gate my lords appear;
Their tinkling bells with measured sound draw near.

How goes the night? I may not slumber now.
The darkness smiles with morning on its brow.
The courtyard torch no more gives forth its ray,
But heralds with its smoke the coming day.
My princes pass the gate, and gather there;
I see their banners floating in the air.

Moral Lessons from Natural Facts

All true words fly, as from yon reedy marsh
The crane rings o'er the wild its screaming harsh.
Vainly you try reason in chains to keep;—
Freely it moves as fish sweeps through the deep.

Hate follows love, as 'neath those sandal-trees
The withered leaves the eager searcher sees.
The hurtful ne'er without some good was born;—
The stones that mar the hill will grind the corn.

All true words spread, as from the marsh's eye
The crane's sonorous note ascends the sky.
Goodness throughout the widest sphere abides,
As fish round isle and through the ocean glides.
And lesser good near greater you shall see,
As grows the paper shrub 'neath sandal-tree.
And good emerges from what man condemns;—
Those stones that mar the hill will polish gems.

BOOK IV

THE DECADE OF K'E-FOO

On the Completion of a Royal Palace

On yonder banks a palace, lo! upshoots,
 The tender blue of southern hill behind;
Firm-founded, like the bamboo's clamping roots;
 Its roof made pine-like, to a point defined.
Fraternal love here bears its precious fruits,
 And unfraternal schemes be ne'er designed!

Ancestral sway is his. The walls they rear,
 Five thousand cubits long; and south and west
The doors are placed. Here will the king appear,
 Here laugh, here talk, here sit him down and rest.

To mould the walls, the frames they firmly tie;
 The toiling builders beat the earth and lime.
The walls shall vermin, storm, and bird defy;—
 Fit dwelling is it for his lordly prime.

Grand is the hall the noble lord ascends;—
 In height, like human form most reverent, grand;
And straight, as flies the shaft when bow unbends;
 Its tints, like hues when pheasant's wings expand.

High pillars rise the level court around;
 The pleasant light the open chamber steeps;
And deep recesses, wide alcoves, are found,
 Where our good king in perfect quiet sleeps.

Laid is the bamboo mat on rush mat square;—
 Here shall he sleep, and, waking, say, "Divine
 What dreams are good? For bear and grizzly bear,
 And snakes and cobras, haunt this couch of mine."

Then shall the chief diviner glad reply,
 "The bears foreshow that Heaven will send you sons.
The snakes and cobras daughters prophesy.
 These auguries are all auspicious ones.

"Sons shall be his—on couches lulled to rest.
 The little ones, enrobed, with sceptres play;
Their infant cries are loud as stern behest;

Their knees the vermeil covers shall display.
As king hereafter one shall be addressed;
The rest, our princes, all the States shall sway.

"And daughters also to him shall be born.
They shall be placed upon the ground to sleep;
Their playthings tiles, their dress the simplest worn;
Their part alike from good and ill to keep,
And ne'er their parents' hearts to cause to mourn;
To cook the food, and spirit-malt to steep."

The Condition of King Seuen's Flocks

Who dares to say your sheep are few?
The flocks are all three hundred strong.
Who dares despise your cattle too?
There ninety, black-lipped, press along.
Though horned the sheep, yet peaceful each appears;
The cattle come with moist and flapping ears.

These climb the heights, those drink the pool;
Some lie at rest, while others roam.
With rain-coats, and thin splint hats cool,
And bearing food, your herdsmen come.
In thirties, ranged by hues, the creatures stand;
Fit victims they will yield at your command.

Your herdsmen twigs and fagots bring,
With prey of birds and beasts for food.
Your sheep, untouched by evil thing,
Approach, their health and vigor good.
The herdsman's waving hand they all behold,
And docile come, and pass into the fold.

Your herdsmen dream;—fish take the place
Of men; on banners falcons fly,
Displacing snakes and tortoises.
The augur tells his prophecy:—
"The first betoken plenteous years; the change
Of banners shows of homes a widening range."

BOOK V

THE DECADE OF SEAOU MIN

A Eunuch Complains of His Fate

A few fine lines, at random drawn,
Like the shell-pattern wrought in lawn
  To hasty glance will seem.
My trivial faults base slander's slime
Distorted into foulest crime,
  And men me worthless deem.

A few small points, pricked down on wood,
May be made out a picture good
  Of the bright Southern Sieve.
Who planned, and helped those slanderers vile,
My name with base lies to defile?
  Unpitied, here I grieve.

With babbling tongues you go about,
And only scheme how to make out
  The lies you scatter round.
Hear me—Be careful what you say;
People ere long your words will weigh,
  And liars you'll be found.

Clever you are with changeful schemes!
How else could all your evil dreams
  And slanders work their way?
Men now believe you; by and by,
The truth found out, each vicious lie
  Will ill for ill repay.

The proud rejoice; the sufferer weeps.
O azure Heaven, from out thy deeps
  Why look in silence down?
Behold those proud men and rebuke;
With pity on the sufferers look,
  And on the evil frown.

Those slanderers I would gladly take,
With all who help their schemes to make,
  And to the tigers throw.
If wolves and tigers such should spare,
Td hurl them 'midst the freezing air,

Where the keen north winds blow.
And should the North compassion feel
I'd fling them to great Heaven, to deal
On them its direst woe.

As on the sacred heights you dwell,
My place is in the willow dell,
One is the other near.
Before you, officers, I spread
These lines by me, poor eunuch, made.
Think not Mang-tsze severe.

An Officer Deplores the Misery of the Time

In the fourth month summer shines;
In the sixth the heat declines.
Nature thus grants men relief;
Tyranny gives only grief.
Were not my forefathers men?
Can my suffering 'scape their ken?

In the cold of autumn days
Each plant shrivels and decays.
Nature then is hard and stern;
Living things sad lessons learn.
Friends dispersed, all order gone,
Place of refuge have I none.

Winter days are wild and fierce;
Rapid gusts each crevice pierce.
Such is my unhappy lot,
Unbefriended and forgot!
Others all can happy be;
I from misery ne'er am free.

On the mountains are fine trees;
Chestnuts, plum-trees, there one sees.
All the year their forms they show;
Stately more and more they grow.
Noble turned to ravening thief!
What the cause? This stirs my grief.

Waters from that spring appear
Sometimes foul, and sometimes clear,
Changing oft as falls the rain,
Or the sky grows bright again.

New misfortunes every day
Still befall me, misery's prey.

Aid from mighty streams obtained,
Southern States are shaped and drained.
Thus the Keang and Han are thanked,
And as benefactors ranked.
Weary toil my vigor drains;
All unnoticed it remains!

Hawks and eagles mount the sky;
Sturgeons in deep waters lie.
Out of reach, they safely get,
Arrow fear not, nor the net.
Hiding-place for me there's none;
Here I stay, and make my moan.

Ferns upon the hills abound; *Ke* and *e* in marshy ground. Each can boast its proper place, Where it grows for use or grace. I can only sing the woe, Which, ill-starred, I undergo.

On the Alienation of a Friend

Gently and soft the east wind blows,
And then there falls the pelting rain.
When anxious fears pressed round you close,
Then linked together were we twain.
Now happy, and your mind at rest,
You turn and cast me from your breast.

Gently and soft the east wind blows,
And then there comes the whirlwind wild.
When anxious fears pressed round you close,
Your bosom held me as a child.
Now happy, and in peaceful state,
You throw me off and quite forget.

Gently and soft the east wind blows,
Then round the rocky height it storms.
Each plant its leaves all dying shows;
The trees display their withered forms.
My virtues great forgotten all,
You keep in mind my faults, though small.

BOOK VI

THE DECADE OF PIH SHAN

A Picture of Husbandry

Various the toils which fields so large demand!
We choose the seed; we take our tools in hand.
In winter for our work we thus prepare;
Then in the spring, bearing the sharpened 'share,
We to the acres go that south incline,
And to the earth the different seeds consign.
Soon, straight and large, upward each plant aspires;—
All happens as our noble lord desires.

The plants will ear; within their sheath confined,
The grains will harden, and be good in kind.
Nor darnel these, nor wolf's-tail grass infests;
From core and leaf we pick the insect pests,
And pick we those that eat the joints and roots:—
So do we guard from harm the growing fruits.
May the great Spirit, whom each farmer names,
Those insects take, and cast them to the flames!

The clouds o'erspread the sky in masses dense,
And gentle rain down to the earth dispense.
First may the public fields the blessing get,
And then with it our private fields we wet!
Patches of unripe grain the reaper leaves;
And here and there ungathered are the sheaves.
Handfuls besides we drop upon the ground,
And ears untouched in numbers lie around;—

These by the poor and widows shall be found.
When wives and children to the toilers come,
Bringing provisions from each separate home,
Our lord of long descent shall oft appear;
The Inspector also, glad the men to cheer.
They too shall thank the Spirits of the air,
With sacrifices pure for all their care;
Now red, now black, the victims that they slay,
As North or South the sacrifice they pay;
While millet bright the altars always show;—
And we shall thus still greater blessings know.

The Complaint of an Officer

O Heaven above, before whose light
Revealed is every deed and thought,
  To thee I cry.
Hither on toilsome service brought,
In this wild K'ew I watch time's flight,
  And sadly sigh.
The second month had just begun,
When from the east we took our way.
  Through summer hot
We passed, and many a wintry day.
Summer again its course has run.
  O bitter lot!
There are my compeers, gay at court,
While here the tears my face begrime.
  I'd fain return—
But there is that dread net for crime!
The fear of it the wish cuts short.
  In vain I burn!

Ere we the royal city left,
The sun and moon renewed the year.
  We marched in hope.
Now to its close this year is near.
Return deferred, of hope bereft,
  All mourn and mope.
My lonesome state haunts aye my breast,
While duties grow, and cares increase,
  Too hard to bear.

Toils that oppress me never cease;
Not for a moment dare I rest,
  Nigh to despair.
I think with fond regard of those,
Who in their posts at court remain,
  My friends of old.
Fain would I be with them again,
But fierce reproof return would cause.
  This post I hold.

When for the West I left my home,
The sun and moon both mildly shone,
  Our hearts to cheer.
We'd soon be back, our service done!
Alas! affairs more urgent come,
  And fix us here.
The year is hastening to expire.
We gather now the southern-wood,

The beans we reap;—
That for its fragrance, these for food.
Such things that constant care require
Me anxious keep.
Thinking of friends still at their posts,
I rise and pass the night outside,
So vexed my mind.
But soon what changes may betide?
I here will stay, whate'er it costs,
And be resigned.

My honored friends, O do not deem
Your rest which seems secure from ill
Will ever last!
Your duties quietly fulfil,
And hold the upright in esteem,
With friendship fast.
So shall the Spirits hear your cry,
You virtuous make, and good supply,
In measure vast.

My honored friends, O do not deem
Repose that seems secure from ill
Will lasting prove.
Your duties quietly fulfil,
And hold the upright in esteem,
With earnest love.
So shall the Spirits hear your prayer,
And on you happiness confer,
Your hopes above.

BOOK VII

DECADE OF SANG HOO

The Rejoicings of a Bridegroom

With axle creaking, all on fire I went,
 To fetch my young and lovely bride.
No thirst or hunger pangs my bosom rent—
 I only longed to have her by my side.
I feast with her, whose virtue fame had told,
Nor need we friends our rapture to behold.

The long-tailed pheasants surest covert find,
 Amid the forest on the plain.
Here from my virtuous bride, of noble mind,
 And person tall, I wisdom gain.
I praise her while we feast, and to her say,
"The love I bear you ne'er will know decay.

"Poor we may be; spirits and viands fine
 My humble means will not afford.
But what we have, we'll taste and not repine;
 From us will come no grumbling word.
And though to you no virtue I can add,
Yet we will sing and dance, in spirit glad.

"I oft ascend that lofty ridge with toil,
 And hew large branches from the oaks;
Then of their leafy glory them I spoil,
 And fagots form with vigorous strokes.
Returning tired, your matchless grace I see,
And my whole soul dissolves in ecstasy.

"To the high hills I looked, and urged each steed;
 The great road next was smooth and plain.

Up hill, o'er dale, I never slackened speed;
 Like lute-string sounded every rein.
I knew, my journey ended, I should come
To you, sweet bride, the comfort of my home."

Against Listening to Slanderers

Like the blueflies buzzing round,
 And on the fences lighting,

Are the sons of slander found,
  Who never cease their biting.
O thou happy, courteous king,
To the winds their slanders fling.

Buzzing round the blueflies hear,
  About the jujubes flocking!
So the slanderers appear,
  Whose calumnies are shocking.
By no law or order bound,
All the kingdom they confound.

How they buzz, those odious flies,
  Upon the hazels clust'ring!
And as odious are the lies
  Of those slanderers blust'ring.
Hatred stirred between us two
Shows the evil they can do.

BOOK VIII

THE DECADE OF TOO JIN SZE

In Praise of By-gone Simplicity

In the old capital they stood,
  With yellow fox-furs plain,
Their manners all correct and good,
  Speech free from vulgar stain.
Could we go back to Chow's old days,
All would look up to them with praise.

In the old capital they wore
  T'ae hats and black caps small;
And ladies, who famed surnames bore,
  Their own thick hair let fall.
Such simple ways are seen no more,
And the changed manners I deplore.

Ear-rings, made of plainest gold,
  In the old days were worn.
Each lady of a noble line
  A Yin or Keih seemed born.
Such officers and ladies now
I see not and my sorrows grow.

With graceful sweep their girdles fell,
  Then in the days of old.
The ladies' side-hair, with a swell,
  Like scorpion's tail, rose bold.
Such, if I saw them in these days,
I'd follow with admiring gaze.

So hung their girdles, not for show;—
  To their own length 'twas due.
'Twas not by art their hair curled so;—
  By nature so it grew.
I seek such manners now in vain,
And pine for them with longing pain.

[NOTE.—Yin and Keih were clan names of great families, the ladies of which would be leaders of fashion in the capital.]

A Wife Bemoans Her Husband's Absence

So full am I of anxious thought,
Though all the morn king-grass I've sought,
  To fill my arms I fail.
Like wisp all-tangled is my hair!
To wash it let me home repair.
  My lord soon may I hail!

Though 'mong the indigo I've wrought
The morning long; through anxious thought
  My skirt's filled but in part.
Within five days he was to appear;
The sixth has come and he's not here.
  Oh! how this racks my heart!

When here we dwelt in union sweet,
If the hunt called his eager feet,
  His bow I cased for him.
Or if to fish he went away,
And would be absent all the day,
  His line I put in trim.

What in his angling did he catch?
Well worth the time it was to watch
  How bream and tench he took.
Men thronged upon the banks and gazed;
At bream and tench they looked amazed,
  The triumphs of his hook.

The Earl of Shaou's Work

As the young millet, by the genial rain
  Enriched, shoots up luxuriant and tall,
So, when we southward marched with toil and pain,
  The Earl of Shaou cheered and inspired us all.

We pushed our barrows, and our burdens bore;
  We drove our wagons, and our oxen led.
"The work once done, our labor there is o'er,
  And home we travel," to ourselves we said.

Close kept our footmen round the chariot track;
  Our eager host in close battalions sped.
"When once our work is done, then we go back,
  Our labor over," to themselves they said.

Hard was the work we had at Seay to do,
  But Shaou's great earl the city soon upreared.
The host its service gave with ardor true;—
  Such power in all the earl's commands appeared!

We did on plains and low lands what was meet;
  We cleared the springs and streams, the land to drain.
The Earl of Shaou announced his work complete,
  And the King's heart reposed, at rest again.

The Plaint of King Yew's Forsaken Wife

The fibres of the white-flowered rush
  Are with the white grass bound.
So do the two together go,
  In closest union found.
And thus should man and wife abide,
  The twain combined in one;
But this bad man sends me away,
  And bids me dwell alone.

Both rush and grass from the bright clouds
  The genial dew partake.

Kind and impartial, nature's laws
  No odious difference make.
But providence appears unkind;
  Events are often hard.
This man, to principle untrue,
  Denies me his regard.

Northward the pools their waters send,
  To flood each paddy field;
So get the fields the sap they need,
  Their store of rice to yield.
But that great man no deed of grace
  Deigns to bestow on me.
My songs are sighs. At thought of him
  My heart aches wearily.

The mulberry branches they collect,
  And use their food to cook;
But I must use a furnace small,
  That pot nor pan will brook.
So me that great man badly treats,
  Nor uses as his wife,

Degrades me from my proper place,
And fills with grief my life.

The bells and drums inside the court
Men stand without and hear;
So should the feelings in my breast,
To him distinct appear.
All-sorrowful, I think of him,
Longing to move his love;
But he vouchsafes no kind response;
His thoughts far from me rove.

The marabow stands on the dam,
And to repletion feeds;
The crane deep in the forest cries,
Nor finds the food it needs.
So in my room the concubine
By the great man is placed;
While I with cruel banishment
Am cast out and disgraced.

The yellow ducks sit on the dam,
With left wing gathered low;
So on each other do they lean,
And their attachment show.
And love should thus the man and wife
In closest concord bind;
But that man turns away from me,
And shows a fickle mind.

When one stands on a slab of stone,
No higher than the ground,
Nothing is added to his height;—
Low with the stone he's found.
So does the favorite's mean estate
Render that great man mean,
While I by him, to distance sent,
Am pierced with sorrow keen.

Hospitality

A few gourd leaves that waved about
Cut down and boiled;—the feast how spare!
But the good host his spirits takes,
Pours out a cup, and proves them rare.

A single rabbit on the mat,
  Or baked, or roast:—how small the feast!
But the good host his spirits takes,
  And fills the cup of every guest.

A single rabbit on the mat,
  Roasted or broiled:—how poor the meal!
But the guests from the spirit vase
  Fill their host's cup, and drink his weal.

A single rabbit on the mat,
  Roasted or baked:—no feast we think!
But from the spirit vase they take,
  Both host and guests, and joyous drink.

On the Misery of Soldiers

Yellow now is all the grass;
All the days in marching pass.
On the move is every man;
Hard work, far and near, they plan.

Black is every plant become;
Every man is torn from home.
Kept on foot, our state is sad;—
As if we no feelings had!

Not rhinoceroses we!
Tigers do we care to be?
Fields like these so desolate
Are to us a hateful fate.

Long-tailed foxes pleased may hide
'Mong the grass, where they abide.
We, in box carts slowly borne,
On the great roads plod and mourn.

PART III.—GREATER ODES OF THE KINGDOM

BOOK I

DECADE OF KING WAN

Celebrating King Wan

The royal Wan now rests on high,
Enshrined in brightness of the sky.
Chow as a state had long been known,
And Heaven's decree at last was shown.
Its lords had borne a glorious name;
God kinged them when the season came.
King Wan ruled well when earth he trod;
Now moves his spirit near to God.

A strong-willed, earnest king was Wan,
And still his fame rolls widening on.
The gifts that God bestowed on Chow
Belong to Wan's descendants now.
Heaven blesses still with gifts divine
The hundred scions of his line;
And all the officers of Chow
From age to age more lustrous grow.

More lustrous still from age to age,
All reverent plans their zeal engage;
And brilliant statesmen owe their birth
To this much-favored spot of earth.
They spring like products of the land—
The men by whom the realm doth stand.
Such aid their numerous bands supply,
That Wan rests tranquilly on high.

Deep were Wan's thoughts, sustained his ways;
His reverence lit its trembling rays.
Resistless came great Heaven's decree;
The sons of Shang must bend the knee;—
The sons of Shang, each one a king,
In numbers beyond numbering.
Yet as God spoke, so must it be:—
The sons of Shang all bent the knee.

Now each to Chow his homage pays—
So dark and changing are Heaven's ways.
When we pour our libations here,
The officers of Shang appear,

Quick and alert to give their aid:—
Such is the service by them paid,
While still they do not cast aside
The cap and broidered axe—their pride.
Ye servants of our line of kings,
Remember him from whom it springs.

Remember him from whom it springs;—
Let this give to your virtue wings.
Seek harmony with Heaven's great mind;—
So shall you surest blessing find.
Ere Shang had lost the nation's heart,
Its monarchs all with God had part
In sacrifice. From them you see
'Tis hard to keep high Heaven's decree.

'Tis hard to keep high Heaven's decree!
O sin not, or you cease to be.
To add true lustre to your name,
See Shang expire in Heaven's dread flame.
For Heaven's high dealings are profound,
And far transcend all sense and sound.
From Wan your pattern you must draw,
And all the States will own your law.

[Book II. is omitted]

BOOK III [*]

DECADE OF TANG

King Seuen on the Occasion of a Great Drought

Grand shone the Milky Way on high,
With brilliant span athwart the sky,
  Nor promise gave of rain.
King Seuen long gazed; then from him broke,
In anguished tones the words he spoke.
  Well might he thus complain!
"O Heaven, what crimes have we to own,
That death and ruin still come down?
Relentless famine fills our graves.
Pity the king who humbly craves!
  Our miseries never cease.
To every Spirit I have vowed;
The choicest victim's blood has flowed.
As offerings I have freely paid
My store of gems and purest jade.
  Hear me, and give release!

"The drought consumes us. As on wing
Its fervors fly, and torment bring.
With purest mind and ceaseless care
My sacrifices I prepare.
At thine own border altars, Heaven,
And in my father's fane, I've given
  What might relief have found.
What Powers above, below, have sway,
To all my precious gifts I pay,
  Then bury in the ground.
Yes, every Spirit has received
Due honor, and, still unrelieved,
  Our sufferings greater grow.
How-tseih can't give the needed aid,
And help from God is still delayed!
The country lies a ruined waste.
O would that I alone might taste
  This bitter cup of woe!

"The drought consumes us. Nor do I
To fix the blame on others try.
I quake with dread; the risk I feel,
As when I hear the thunders peal,
  Or fear its sudden crash.

Our black-haired race, a remnant now,
Will every one be swept from Chow,
  As by the lightning's flash.
Nor I myself will live alone.
God from his great and heavenly throne
  Will not spare even me.
O friends and officers, come, blend
Your prayers with mine; come, lowly bend.
Chow's dynasty will pass away;
Its altars at no distant day
  In ruins all shall be!

"The drought consumes us. It keeps on
Its fatal course. All hope is gone.
The air more fierce and fiery glows.
Where can I fly? Where seek repose?
  Death marks me for its prey.
Above, no saving hand! Around,
No hope, no comfort, can be found.
The dukes and ministers of old
Give us no help. Can ye withhold
Your sympathy, who lately reigned?
And parents, how are you restrained,
  In this so dreadful day?

"The drought consumes us. There on high
The hills are parched. The streams are dry.
Drought's demon stalks abroad in ire,
And scatters wide his flames and fire.
  Alas, my woful heart!
The fires within its strength consume;
The heat without creates a gloom
  That from it will not part.
The dukes and ministers by-gone
Respond not to my prayer and moan.
God in great Heaven, permission give
That I may in retirement live,
  And try to heal my smart!

"The drought consumes us. Still I strive,
And will not leave while I survive.
  Duty to shun I fear.
Why upon me has come this drought?
Vainly I try to search it out,
  Vainly, with quest severe.
For a good harvest soon I prayed,
Nor late the rites I duly paid,

To Spirits of the air and land.
There wanted nought they could demand,
  Their favor to secure.
God in great heaven, be just, be kind!
Thou dost not bear me in Thy mind.
My cry, ye wisest Spirits, hear!
Ye whom I constantly revere,
  Why do I this endure?

"The drought consumes us. People fly,
And leave their homes. Each social tie
  And bond of rule is snapt.
The Heads of Boards are all perplexed;
My premier's mind is sorely vexed;
  In trouble all are wrapt.
The Masters of my Horse and Guards;
My cook, and men of different wards:—
Not one has from the struggle shrunk.
Though feeling weak, they have not sunk,
  But done their best to aid.
To the great sky I look with pain;—
Why do these grievous sorrows rain
  On my devoted head?

"Yes, at the mighty sky I gaze,
And lo! the stars pursue their maze,
  And sparkle clear and bright.
Ah! Heaven nor helps, nor seems to ken.
Great officers and noble men,
With all your powers ye well have striven,
And reverently have sought from Heaven
  Its aid in our great fight.
My death is near; but oh! keep on,
And do as thus far you have done.
  Regard you only me?
No, for yourselves and all your friends,
On whom for rule the land depends,
  You seek security.
I turn my gaze to the great sky;—
When shall this drought be done, and I
  Quiet and restful be?"

[NOTE *: Selections from Book II. are omitted.—EDITOR.]

PART IV.—ODES OF THE TEMPLE AND ALTAR

BOOK I

SACRIFICIAL ODES OF CHOW

Appropriate to a Sacrifice to King Wan

My offerings here are given,
  A ram, a bull.
Accept them, mighty Heaven,
  All-bountiful.

Thy statutes, O great king,
  I keep, I love;
So on the realm to bring
  Peace from above.

From Wan comes blessing rich;
  Now on the right
He owns those gifts to which
  Him I invite.

Do I not night and day,
  Revere great Heaven,
That thus its favor may
  To Chow be given?

On Sacrificing to the Kings Woo, Ching, and K'ang

The arm of Woo was full of might;
  None could his fire withstand;
And Ching and K'ang stood forth to sight,
  As kinged by God's own hand.

We err not when we call them sage.
  How grandly they maintained
Their hold of all the heritage
  That Wan and Woo had gained!

As here we worship, they descend,
  While bells and drums resound,
And stones and lutes their music blend.
  With blessings we are crowned.

The rites correctly we discharge;
  The feast we freely share.

Those Sires Chow's glory will enlarge,
And ever for it care.

THE TRAVELS OF FA-HIEN

[Translation by James Legge]

TRANSLATOR'S INTRODUCTION

Nothing of great importance is known about Fa-hien in addition to what may be gathered from his own record of his travels. I have read the accounts of him in the "Memoirs of Eminent Monks," compiled in A.D. 519, and a later work, the "Memoirs of Marvellous Monks," by the third emperor of the Ming dynasty (A.D. 1403-1424), which, however, is nearly all borrowed from the other; and all in them that has an appearance of verisimilitude can be brought within brief compass.

His surname, they tell us, was Kung, and he was a native of Wu-yang in P'ing-yang, which is still the name of a large department in Shan-hsi. He had three brothers older than himself; but when they all died before shedding their first teeth, his father devoted him to the service of the Buddhist society, and had him entered as a Sramanera, still keeping him at home in the family. The little fellow fell dangerously ill, and the father sent him to the monastery, where he soon got well and refused to return to his parents.

When he was ten years old, his father died; and an uncle, considering the widowed solitariness and helplessness of the mother, urged him to renounce the monastic life, and return to her, but the boy replied, "I did not quit the family in compliance with my father's wishes, but because I wished to be far from the dust and vulgar ways of life. This is why I choose monkhood." The uncle approved of his words and gave over urging him. When his mother also died, it appeared how great had been the affection for her of his fine nature; but after her burial he returned to the monastery.

On one occasion he was cutting rice with a score or two of his fellow-disciples, when some hungry thieves came upon them to take away their grain by force. The other Sramaneras all fled, but our young hero stood his ground, and said to the thieves, "If you must have the grain, take what you please. But, sirs, it was your former neglect of charity which brought you to your present state of destitution; and now, again, you wish to rob others. I am afraid that in the coming ages you will have still greater poverty and distress; I am sorry for you beforehand." With these words he followed his companions to the monastery, while the thieves left the grain and went away, all the monks, of whom there were several hundred, doing homage to his conduct and courage.

When he had finished his novitiate and taken on him the obligations of the full Buddhist orders, his earnest courage, clear intelligence, and strict regulation of his demeanor, were conspicuous; and soon after, he undertook his journey to India in search of complete copies of the Vinaya-pitaka. What follows this is merely an account of his travels in India and return to China by sea, condensed from his own narrative, with the addition of some marvellous incidents that happened to him, on his visit to the Vulture Peak near Rajagriha.

It is said in the end that after his return to China, he went to the capital (evidently Nanking), and there, along with the Indian Sramana Buddha-bhadra, executed translations of some of the works which he had obtained in India; and that before he had done all that he wished to do in this way, he removed to King-chow (in the present Hoo-pih), and died in the monastery of Sin, at the age of eighty-eight, to the great sorrow of all who knew him. It is added that there is another larger work giving an account of his travels in various countries.

Such is all the information given about our author, beyond what he has himself told us. Fa-hien was his clerical name, and means "Illustrious in the Law," or "Illustrious master of the Law." The Shih which often precedes it is an abbreviation of the name of Buddha as Sakyamuni, "the Sakya, mighty in Love, dwelling in Seclusion and Silence," and may be taken as equivalent to Buddhist. He is sometimes said to have belonged to "the eastern Tsin dynasty" (A.D. 317-419), and sometimes to "the Sung," that is, the Sung dynasty of the House of Liu (A.D. 420-478). If he became a full monk at the age of twenty, and went to India when he was twenty-five, his long life may have been divided pretty equally between the two dynasties.

If there were ever another and larger account of Fa-hien's travels than the narrative of which a translation is now given, it has long ceased to be in existence.

In the catalogue of the imperial library of the Suy dynasty (A.D. 589-618), the name Fa-hien occurs four times. Towards the end of the last section of it, after a reference to his travels, his labors in translation at Kin-ling (another name for Nanking), in conjunction with Buddha-bhadra, are described. In the second section we find "A Record of Buddhistic Kingdoms"—with a note, saying that it was the work of "the Sramana, Fa-hien"; and again, we have "Narrative of Fa-hien in two Books," and "Narrative of Fa-hien's Travels in one Book." But all these three entries may possibly belong to different copies of the same work, the first and the other two being in separate subdivisions of the catalogue.

In the two Chinese copies of the narrative in my possession the title is "Record of Buddhistic Kingdoms." In the Japanese or Corean recension the title is twofold; first, "Narrative of the Distinguished Monk, Fa-hien"; and then, more at large, "Incidents of Travels in India, by the Sramana of the Eastern Tsin, Fa-hien, recorded by himself."

There is still earlier attestation of the existence of our little work than the Suy catalogue. The "Catalogue Raisonne" of the imperial library of the present dynasty mentions two quotations from it by Le Tao-yueen, a geographical writer of the dynasty of the Northern Wei (A.D. 386-584), one of them containing eighty-nine characters, and the other two hundred and seventy-six; both of them given as from the "Narrative of Fa-hien."

In all catalogues subsequent to that of Suy our work appears. The evidence for its authenticity and genuineness is all that could be required. It is clear to myself that the "Record of Buddhistic Kingdoms" and the "Narrative of his Travels by Fa-hien" were designations of one and the same work, and that it is doubtful whether any larger work on the same subject was ever current. With regard to the text subjoined to my translation, it was published in Japan in 1779. The editor had before him four recensions of the narrative; those of the Sung and Ming dynasties, with appendices on the names of certain characters in them; that of Japan; and that of Corea. He wisely adopted the Corean text, published in accordance with a royal rescript in 1726, so far as I can make out; but the different readings of the other texts are all given in top-notes, instead of foot-notes as with us, this being one of the points in which customs in the East and West go by contraries. Very occasionally, the editor indicates by a single character, equivalent to "right" or "wrong," which reading in his opinion is to be preferred.

The editors of the "Catalogue Raisonne" intimate their doubts of the good taste and reliability of all Fa-hien's statements. It offends them that he should call central India the "Middle Kingdom," and China, which to them was the true and only Middle Kingdom, but "a Border-land"—it offends them as the vaunting language of a Buddhist writer, whereas the reader will see in the expressions only an instance of what Fa-hien calls his "simple straightforwardness."

As an instance of his unreliability they refer to his account of the Buddhism of Khoten, whereas it is well-known, they say, that the Khoteners from ancient times till now have been Mohammedans;—as if they could have been so one hundred and seventy years before Mohammed was born, and two hundred twenty-two years before the year of the Hegira! And this is criticism in China. The catalogue was ordered by the K'ien-lung emperor in 1722. Between three and four hundred of the "Great Scholars" of the empire were engaged on it in various departments, and thus egregiously ignorant did they show themselves of all beyond the limits of their own country, and even of the literature of that country itself.

Much of what Fa-hien tells his readers of Buddhist miracles and legends is indeed unreliable and grotesque; but we have from him the truth as to what he saw and heard.

In concluding this introduction I wish to call attention to some estimates of the number of Buddhists in the world which have become current, believing, as I do, that the smallest of them is much above what is correct.

In a note on the first page of his work on the Bhilsa Topes (1854), General Cunningham says: "The Christians number about two hundred and seventy millions; the Buddhists about two hundred and twenty-two millions, who are distributed as follows: China one hundred and seventy millions, Japan twenty-five millions, Anam fourteen millions, Siam three millions, Ava eight millions, Népal one million, and Ceylon one million." In his article on M.J. Barthelemy Saint-Hilaire's "Le Bouddha et sa Religion," republished in his "Chips from a German workshop," vol. i. (1868), Professor Max Mueller says, "The young prince became the founder of a religion which, after more than two thousand years, is still professed by four hundred and fifty-five millions of human beings," and he appends the following note: "Though truth is not settled by majorities, it would be interesting to know which religion counts at the present moment the largest numbers of believers. Berghaus, in his 'Physical Atlas,' gives the following division of the human race according to religion: 'Buddhists 31.2 per cent., Christians 30.7, Mohammedans 15.7, Brahmanists 13.4, Heathens 8.7, and Jews O.3.' As Berghaus does not distinguish the Buddhists in China from the followers of Confucius and Laotse, the first place on the scale belongs really to Christianity. It is difficult in China to say to what religion a man belongs, as the same person may profess two or three. The emperor himself, after sacrificing according to the ritual of Confucius, visits a Tao-tse temple, and afterwards bows before an image of Fo in a Buddhist chapel." ("Melanges Asiatiques de St. Petersbourg," vol. ii. p. 374.)

Both these estimates are exceeded by Dr. T.W. Rhys Davids (intimating also the uncertainty of the statements, and that numbers are no evidence of truth) in the introduction to his "Manual of Buddhism." The Buddhists there appear as amounting in all to five hundred millions:—thirty millions of Southern Buddhists, in Ceylon, Burma, Siam, Anam, and India (Jains); and four hundred and seventy millions of Northern Buddhists, of whom nearly thirty-three millions are assigned to Japan, and 414,686,974 to the eighteen provinces of China proper. According to him, Christians amount to about 26 per cent, of mankind, Hindus to about 13, Mohammedans to about 12-1/2, Buddhists to about 40, and Jews to about one-half of one per cent.

In regard to all these estimates, it will be observed that the immense numbers assigned to Buddhism are made out by the multitude of Chinese with which it is credited. Subtract Cunningham's one hundred and seventy millions of Chinese from his total of two hundred and twenty-two millions, and there remain only fifty-two millions of Buddhists. Subtract Davids's four hundred fourteen and one-half millions of Chinese from his total of five hundred millions, and there remain only eighty-five and one-half millions for Buddhism. Of the numbers assigned to other countries, as well as of their whole populations, I am in considerable doubt, excepting in the cases of Ceylon and India; but the greatness of the estimates turns upon the immense multitudes said to be in China. I do not know what total population Cunningham allowed for that country, nor on what principle he allotted one hundred and seventy millions of it to Buddhism; perhaps he halved his estimate of the whole, whereas Berghaus and Davids allotted to it the highest estimates that have been given of the people.

But we have no certain information of the population of China. At an interview with the former Chinese ambassador, Kwo Sung-tao, in Paris, in 1878, I begged him to write out for me the amount, with the authority for it, and he assured me that it could not be done. I have read probably almost everything that has been published on the subject, and endeavored by methods of my own to arrive at a satisfactory conclusion;—without reaching a result which I can venture to lay before the public. My impression has been that four hundred millions is hardly an exaggeration.

But supposing that we had reliable returns of the whole population, how shall we proceed to apportion that among Confucianists, Taoists, and Buddhists? Confucianism is the orthodoxy of China. The common name for it is Ju Chiao, "the Doctrines held by the Learned Class," entrance into the circle of which is, with a few insignificant exceptions, open to all the people. The mass of them and the masses under their influence are preponderatingly Confucian; and in the observance of ancestral worship, the most remarkable feature of the religion proper of China from the earliest times, of which Confucius was not the author but the prophet, an overwhelming majority are regular and assiduous.

Among "the strange principles" which the emperor of the K'ang-hsi period, in one of his famous Sixteen Precepts, exhorted his people to "discountenance and put away, in order to exalt the correct doctrine," Buddhism and Taoism were both included. If, as stated in the note quoted from Professor Mueller, the emperor countenances both the Taoist worship and the Buddhist, he does so for reasons of state; to please especially his Buddhistic subjects in Thibet and Mongolia, and not to offend the many whose superstitious fancies incline to Taoism.

When I went out and in as a missionary among the Chinese people for about thirty years, it sometimes occurred to me that only the inmates of their monasteries and the recluses of both systems should be enumerated as Buddhists and Taoists; but I was in the end constrained to widen that judgment, and to admit a considerable following of both among the people, who have neither received the tonsure nor assumed the yellow top. Dr. Eitel, in concluding his discussion of this point in his "Lecture on Buddhism, an Event in History," says: "It is not too much to say that most Chinese are theoretically Confucianists, but emotionally Buddhists or Taoists. But fairness requires us to add that, though the mass of the people are more or less influenced by Buddhist doctrines, yet the people, as a whole, have no respect for the Buddhist church, and habitually sneer at Buddhist priests." For the "most" in the former of these two sentences I would substitute "nearly all;" and between my friend's "but" and "emotionally" I would introduce "many are," and would not care to contest his conclusion further. It does seem to me preposterous to credit Buddhism with the whole of the vast population of China, the great majority of whom are Confucianists. My own opinion is that its adherents are not so many as those even of Mohammedanism, and that instead of being the most numerous of the religions (so-called) of the world, it is only entitled to occupy the fifth place, ranking below Christianity, Confucianism, Brahmanism, and Mohammedanism, and followed, some distance off, by Taoism. To make a table of percentages of mankind, and to assign to each system its proportion, are to seem to be wise where we are deplorably ignorant; and, moreover, if our means of information were much better than they are, our figures would merely show the outward adherence. A fractional percentage might tell more for one system than a very large integral one for another.

JAMES LEGGE.

THE TRAVELS OF FA-HIEN

CHAPTER I

From Ch'ang-gan to the Sandy Desert

Fa-Hien had been living in Ch'ang-gan. [1] Deploring the mutilated and imperfect state of the collection of the Books of Discipline, in the second year of the period Hwang-che, being the Ke-hae year of the cycle, [2] he entered into an engagement with Hwuy-king, Tao-ching, Hwuy-ying, and Hwuy-wei, that they should go to India and seek for the Disciplinary Rules.

After starting from Ch'ang-gan, they passed through Lung, [3] and came to the kingdom of K'een-kwei,[4] where they stopped for the summer retreat. When that was over, they went forward to the kingdom of Now-t'an, crossed the mountain of Yang-low, and reached the emporium of Chang-yih.[5] There they found the country so much disturbed that travelling on the roads was impossible for them. Its king, however, was very attentive to them, kept them in his capital, and acted the part of their danapati.[6]

Here they met with Che-yen, Hwuy-keen, Sang-shao, Pao-yun, and Sang-king; and in pleasant association with them, as bound on the same journey with themselves, they passed the summer retreat of that year [7] together, resuming after it their travelling, and going on to T'un-hwang, [8] the chief town in the frontier territory of defence extending for about eighty li from east to west, and about forty from north to south. Their company, increased as it had been, halted there for some days more than a month, after which Fa-hien and his four friends started first in the suite of an envoy, having separated for a time from Pao-yun and his associates.

Le Hao, the prefect of Tun-hwang, had supplied them with the means of crossing the desert before them, in which there are many evil demons and hot winds. Travellers who encounter them perish all to a man. There is not a bird to be seen in the air above, nor an animal on the ground below. Though you look all round most earnestly to find where you can cross, you know not where to make your choice, the only mark and indication being the dry bones of the dead left upon the sand.

[Footnote 1: Ch'ang-gan is still the name of the principal district (and its city) in the department of Se-gan, Shen-se. It had been the capital of the first empire of Han (B.C. 202 A.D. 24), as it subsequently was that of Suy (A.D. 589-618).]

[Footnote 2: The period Hwang-che embraced from A.D. 399 to 414, being the greater portion of the reign of Yao Hing of the After Ts'in, a powerful prince. He adopted Hwang-che for the style of his reign in 399, and the cyclical name of that year was Kang-tsze. It is not possible at this distance of time to explain, if it could be explained, how Fa-hien came to say that Ke-hae was the second year of the period. It seems most reasonable to suppose that he set out on his pilgrimage in A.D. 399, the cycle name of which was Ke-hae. In the "Memoirs of Eminent Monks" it is said that our author started in the third year of the period Lung-gan of the Eastern Ts'in, which was A.D. 399.]

[Footnote 3: Lung embraced the western part of Shen-se and the eastern part of Kan-suh. The name remains in Lung Chow, in the extreme west of Shen-se.]

[Footnote 4: K'een-kwei was the second king of "the Western Ts'in." Fa-hien would find him at his capital, somewhere in the present department of Lan-chow, Kan-suh.]

[Footnote 5: Chang-yih is still the name of a district in Kan-chow department, Kan-suh. It is a long way north and west from Lan-chow, and not far from the Great Wall. Its king at this time was, probably, Twan-yeh of "the northern Leang."]

[Footnote 6: Dana is the name for religious charity, the first of the six paramitas, or means of attaining to nirvana; and a danapati is "one who practises dana and thereby crosses the sea of misery."]

[Footnote 7: This was the second summer since the pilgrims left Ch'ang-gan. We are now, therefore, probably, in A.D. 400.]

[Footnote 8: T'un-hwang is still the name of one of the two districts constituting the department of Gan-se, the most western of the prefectures of Kan-suh; beyond the termination of the Great Wall.]

CHAPTER II

On to Shen-shen and thence to Khoten

After travelling for seventeen days, a distance we may calculate of about 1500 li, the pilgrims reached the kingdom of Shen-shen, a country rugged and hilly, with a thin and barren soil. The clothes of the common people are coarse, and like those worn in our land of Han, [1] some wearing felt and others coarse serge or cloth of hair; this was the only difference seen among them. The king professed our Law, and there might be in the country more than four thousand monks, who were all students of the hinayana. [2] The common people of this and other kingdoms in that region, as well as the Sramans, [3] all practise the rules of India, only that the latter do so more exactly, and the former more loosely. So the travellers found it in all the kingdoms through which they went on their way from this to the west, only that each had its own peculiar barbarous speech. The monks, however, who had given up the worldly life and quitted their families, were all students of Indian books and the Indian language. Here they stayed for about a month, and then proceeded on their journey, fifteen days' walking to the northwest bringing them to the country of Woo-e. In this also there were more than four thousand monks, all students of the hinayana. They were very strict in their rules, so that Sramans from the territory of Ts'in were all unprepared for their regulations. Fa-hien, through the management of Foo Kung-sun, *maitre d'hotellerie*, was able to remain with his company in the monastery where they were received for more than two months, and here they were rejoined by Pao-yun and his friends. At the end of that time the people of Woo-e neglected the duties of propriety and righteousness, and treated the strangers in so niggardly a manner that Che-yen, Hwuy-keen, and Hwuy-wei went back towards Kao-ch'ang, hoping to obtain there the means of continuing their journey. Fa-hien and the rest, however, through the liberality of Foo Kung-sun, managed to go straight forward in a southwest direction. They found the country uninhabited as they went along. The difficulties which they encountered in crossing the streams and on their route, and the sufferings which they endured, were unparalleled in human experience, but in the course of a month and five days they succeeded in reaching Yu-teen.

[Footnote 1: This is the name which Fa-hien always uses when he would speak of China, his native country, as a whole, calling it from the great dynasty which had ruled it, first and last, for between four and five centuries. Occasionally, as we shall immediately see, he speaks of "the territory of Ts'in or Ch'in," but intending thereby only the kingdom of Ts'in, having its capital in Ch'ang-gan.]

[Footnote 2: Meaning the "small vehicle, or conveyance." There are in Buddhism the triyana, or "three different means of salvation, *i.e.* of conveyance across the samsara, or sea of transmigration, to the shores of nirvana. Afterwards the term was used to designate the different phases of development through which the Buddhist dogma passed, known as the mahayana, hinayana, and madhyamayana." "The hinayana is the simplest vehicle of salvation, corresponding to the first of the three degrees of saintship." E.H., pp. 151-2, 45, and 117.]

[Footnote 3: "Sraman" may in English take the place of Sramana, the name for Buddhist monks, as those who have separated themselves from (left) their families, and quieted their hearts from all intrusion of desire and lust.]

CHAPTER III

Khoten—Processions of Images

Yu-Teen is a pleasant and prosperous kingdom, with a numerous and flourishing population. The inhabitants all profess our Law, and join together in its religious music for their enjoyment. The monks amount to several myriads, most of whom are students of the mahayana. [1] They all receive their food from the common store. Throughout the country the houses of the people stand apart like separate stars, and each family has a small tope [2] reared in front of its door. The smallest of these may be twenty cubits high, or rather more. They make in the monasteries rooms for monks from all quarters, the use of which is given to travelling monks who may arrive, and who are provided with whatever else they require.

The lord of the country lodged Fa-hien and the others comfortably, and supplied their wants, in a monastery called Gomati, of the mahayana school. Attached to it there are three thousand monks, who are called to their meals by the sound of a bell. When they enter the refectory, their demeanor is marked by a reverent gravity, and they take their seats in regular order, all maintaining a perfect silence. No sound is heard from their alms-bowls and other utensils. When any of these pure men require food, they are not allowed to call out to the attendants for it, but only make signs with their hands.

Hwuy-king, Tao-ching, and Hwuy-tah set out in advance towards the country of K'eeh-ch'a; but Fa-hien and the others, wishing to see the procession of images, remained behind for three months. There are in this country four great monasteries, not counting the smaller ones. Beginning on the first day of the fourth month, they sweep and water the streets inside the city, making a grand display in the lanes and byways. Over the city gate they pitch a large tent, grandly adorned in all possible ways, in which the king and queen, with their ladies brilliantly arrayed, take up their residence for the time.

The monks of the Gomati monastery, being mahayana students, and held in greatest reverence by the king, took precedence of all the others in the procession. At a distance of three or four li from the city, they made a four-wheeled image car, more than thirty cubits high, which looked like the great hall of a monastery moving along. The seven precious substances [3] were grandly displayed about it, with silken streamers and canopies hanging all around. The chief image stood in the middle of the car, with two Bodhisattvas [4] in attendance on it, while devas were made to follow in waiting, all brilliantly carved in gold and silver, and hanging in the air. When the car was a hundred paces from the gate, the king put off his crown of state, changed his dress for a fresh suit, and with bare feet, carrying in his hands flowers and incense, and with two rows of attending followers, went out at the gate to meet the image; and, with his head and face bowed to the ground, he did homage at its feet, and then scattered the flowers and burnt the incense. When the image was entering the gate, the queen and the brilliant ladies with her in the gallery above scattered far and wide all kinds of flowers, which floated about and fell promiscuously to the ground. In this way everything was done to promote the dignity of the occasion. The carriages of the monasteries were all different, and each one had its own day for the procession. The ceremony began on the first day of the fourth month, and ended on the fourteenth, after which the king and queen returned to the palace.

Seven or eight li to the west of the city there is what is called the King's new monastery, the building of which took eighty years, and extended over three reigns. It may be two hundred and fifty cubits in height, rich in elegant carving and inlaid work, covered above with gold and silver, and finished throughout with a combination of all the precious substances. Behind the tope there has been built a Hall of Buddha, of the utmost magnificence and beauty, the beams, pillars, venetianed doors and windows, being all overlaid with gold-leaf. Besides this, the apartments for the monks are imposingly and elegantly decorated, beyond the power of words to express. Of whatever things of highest value and preciousness the kings in the six countries on the east of the Ts'ung range of mountains are possessed, they contribute the greater portion to this monastery, using but a small portion of them themselves.

[Footnote 1: Mahayana is a later form of the Buddhist doctrine, the second phase of its development corresponding to the state of a Bodhisattva, who, being able to transport himself and all mankind to nirvana, may be compared to a huge vehicle.]

[Footnote 2: A worshipping place, an altar, or temple.]

[Footnote 3: The Sapta-ratna, gold, silver, lapis lazuli, rock crystal, rubies, diamonds or emeralds, and agate.]

[Footnote 4: A Bodhisattva is one whose essence has become intelligence; a Being who will in some future birth as a man (not necessarily or usually the next) attain to Buddhahood. The name does not include those Buddhas who have not yet attained to parinirvana. The symbol of the state is an elephant fording a river.]

CHAPTER IV

Through the Ts'ung Mountains to K'eech-ch'a

When the processions of images in the fourth month were over, Sang-shao, by himself alone, followed a Tartar who was an earnest follower of the Law, and proceeded towards Ko-phene. Fa-hien and the others went forward to the kingdom of Tsze-hoh, which it took them twenty-five days to reach. Its king was a strenuous follower of our Law, and had around him more than a thousand monks, mostly students of the mahayana. Here the travellers abode fifteen days, and then went south for four days, when they found themselves among the Ts'ung-ling mountains, and reached the country of Yu-hwuy, where they halted and kept their retreat. [1] When this was over, they went on among the hills for twenty-five days, and got to K'eeh-ch'a, there rejoining Hwuy-king and his two companions.

[Footnote 1: This was the retreat already twice mentioned as kept by the pilgrims in the summer, the different phraseology, "quiet rest," without any mention of the season, indicating their approach to India. Two, if not three, years had elapsed since they left Ch'ang-gan. Are we now with them in 402?]

CHAPTER V

Great Quinquennial Assembly of Monks

It happened that the king of the country was then holding the pancha parishad; that is, in Chinese, the great quinquennial assembly. When this is to be held, the king requests the presence of the Sramans from all quarters of his kingdom. They come as if in clouds; and when they are all assembled, their place of session is grandly decorated. Silken streamers and canopies are hung out in it, and water-lilies in gold and silver are made and fixed up behind the places where the chief of them are to sit. When clean mats have been spread, and they are all seated, the king and his ministers present their offerings according to rule and law. The assembly takes place in the first, second, or third month, for the most part in the spring.

After the king has held the assembly, he further exhorts the ministers to make other and special offerings. The doing of this extends over one, two, three, five, or even seven days; and when all is finished, he takes his own riding-horse, saddles, bridles, and waits on him himself, while he makes the noblest and most important minister of the kingdom mount him. Then, taking fine white woollen cloth, all sorts of precious things, and articles which the Sramans require, he distributes them among them, uttering vows at the same time along with all his ministers; and when this distribution has taken place, he again redeems whatever he wishes from the monks.

The country, being among the hills and cold, does not produce the other cereals, and only the wheat gets ripe. After the monks have received their annual portion of this, the mornings suddenly show the hoar-frost, and on this account the king always begs the monks to make the wheat ripen [1] before they receive their portion. There is in the country a spittoon which belonged to Buddha, made of stone, and in color like his alms-bowl. There is also a tooth of Buddha, for which the people have reared a tope, connected with which there are more than a thousand monks and their disciples, all students of the hinayana. To the east of these hills the dress of the common people is of coarse materials, as in our country of Ts'in, but here also there were among them the differences of fine woollen cloth and of serge or haircloth. The rules observed by the Sramans are remarkable, and too numerous to be mentioned in detail. The country is in the midst of the Onion range. As you go forward from these mountains, the plants, trees, and fruits are all different from those of the land of Han, excepting only the bamboo, pomegranate, and sugarcane.

[Footnote 1: Watters calls attention to this as showing that the monks of K'eeh-ch'a had the credit of possessing weather-controlling powers.]

CHAPTER VI

North India—Image of Maitreya Bodhisattva

From this the travellers went westward towards North India, and after being on the way for a month, they succeeded in getting across and through the range of the Onion mountains. The snow rests on them both winter and summer. There are also among them venomous dragons, which, when provoked, spit forth poisonous winds, and cause showers of snow and storms of sand and gravel. Not one in ten thousand of those who encounter these dangers escapes with his life. The people of the country call the range by the name of "The Snow mountains." When the travellers had got through them, they were in North India, and immediately on entering its borders, found themselves in a small kingdom called T'oleih, where also there were many monks, all students of the hinayana.

In this kingdom there was formerly an Arhan, [1] who by his supernatural power took a clever artificer up to the Tushita [2] heaven, to see the height, complexion, and appearance of Maitreya Bodhisattva, [3] and then return and make an image of him in wood. First and last, this was done three times, and then the image was completed, eighty cubits in height, and eight cubits at the base from knee to knee of the crossed legs. On fast-days it emits an effulgent light. The kings of the surrounding countries vie with one another in presenting offerings to it. Here it is—to be seen now as of old.

[Footnote 1: Lo-han, Arhat, Arahat are all designations of the perfected Arya, the disciple who has passed the different stages of the Noble Path, or eightfold excellent way, who has conquered all passions, and is not to be reborn again. Arhatship implies possession of certain supernatural powers, and is not to be succeeded by Buddhaship, but implies the fact of the saint having already attained Nirvana.]

[Footnote 2: Tushita is the fourth Devaloka, where all Bodhisattvas are reborn before finally appearing on earth as Buddha. Life lasts in Tushita four thousand years, but twenty-four hours there are equal to four hundred years on earth.]

[Footnote 3: Maitreya was a Bodhisattva, the principal one, indeed, of Sakyamuni's retinue, but is not counted among the ordinary disciples, nor is anything told of his antecedents. It was in the Tushita heaven that Sakyamuni met him and appointed him as his successor, to appear as Buddha after the lapse of five thousand years. Maitreya is therefore the expected Messiah of the Buddhists, residing at present in Tushita.]

CHAPTER VII

The Perilous Crossing of the Indus

The travellers went on to the southwest for fifteen days at the foot of the mountains, and following the course of their range. The way was difficult and rugged, running along a bank exceedingly precipitous, which rose up there, a hill-like wall of rock, ten thousand cubits from the base. When one approached the edge of it, his eyes became unsteady; and if he wished to go forward in the same direction, there was no place on which he could place his foot; and beneath were the waters of the river called the Indus. In former times men had chiselled paths along the rocks, and distributed ladders on the face of them, to the number altogether of seven hundred, at the bottom of which there was a suspension bridge of ropes, by which the river was crossed, its banks being there eighty paces apart. The place and arrangements are to be found in the Records of the Nine Interpreters, but neither Chang K'een [1] nor Kan Ying [2] had reached the spot.

The monks asked Fa-hien if it could be known when the Law of Buddha first went to the east. He replied, "When I asked the people of those countries about it, they all said that it had been handed down by their fathers from of old that, after the setting up of the image of Maitreya Bodhisattva, there were Sramans of India who crossed this river, carrying with them Sutras and Books of Discipline. Now the image was set up rather more than three hundred years after the Nirvana of Buddha, which may be referred to the reign of king P'ing of the Chow dynasty. According to this account we may say that the diffusion of our great doctrines in the East began from the setting up of this image. If it had not been through that Maitreya, the great spiritual master who is to be the successor of the Sakya, who could have caused the 'Three Precious Ones,' [3] to be proclaimed so far, and the people of those border lands to know our Law? We know of a truth that the opening of the way for such a mysterious propagation is not the work of man; and so the dream of the emperor Ming of Han had its proper cause."

[Footnote 1: Chang K'een, a minister of the emperor Woo of Han (B.C. 140-87), is celebrated as the first Chinese who "pierced the void," and penetrated to "the regions of the west," corresponding very much to the present Turkestan. Through him, by B.C. 115, a regular intercourse was established between China and the thirty-six kingdoms or states of that quarter.]

[Footnote 2: Less is known of Kan Ying than of Chang K'een. Being sent in A.D. 88 by his patron Pan Chao on an embassy to the Roman empire, he only got as far as the Caspian sea, and returned to China. He extended, however, the knowledge of his countrymen with regard to the western regions.]

[Footnote 3: "The precious Buddha," "the precious Law," and "the precious Monkhood"; Buddha, Dharma, and Sangha; the whole being equivalent to Buddhism.]

CHAPTER VIII

Woo-chang, or Udyana—Traces of Buddha

After crossing the river, the travellers immediately came to the kingdom of Woo-chang, which is indeed a part of North India. The people all use the language of Central India, "Central India" being what we should call the "Middle Kingdom." The food and clothes of the common people are the same as in that Central Kingdom. The Law of Buddha is very flourishing in Woo-chang. They call the places where the monks stay for a time or reside permanently Sangharamas; and of these there are in all five hundred, the monks being all students of the hinayana. When stranger bhikshus [1] arrive at one of them, their wants are supplied for three days, after which they are told to find a resting-place for themselves.

There is a tradition that when Buddha came to North India, he came at once to this country, and that here he left a print of his foot, which is long or short according to the ideas of the beholder on the subject. It exists, and the same thing is true about it, at the present day. Here also are still to be seen the rock on which he dried his clothes, and the place where he converted the wicked dragon. The rock is fourteen cubits high, and more than twenty broad, with one side of it smooth.

Hwuy-king, Hwuy-tah, and Tao-ching went on ahead towards the place of Buddha's shadow in the country of Nagara; but Fa-hien and the others remained in Woo-chang, and kept the summer retreat. That over, they descended south, and arrived in the country of Soo-ho-to.

[Footnote 1: Bhikshu is the name for a monk as "living by alms," a mendicant. All bhikshus call themselves Sramans. Sometimes the two names are used together by our author.]

CHAPTER IX

Soo-ho-to—Legends of Buddha

In that country also Buddhism is flourishing. There is in it the place where Sakra, [1] Ruler of Devas, in a former age, tried the Bodhisattva, by producing a hawk in pursuit of a dove, when the Bodhisattva cut off a piece of his own flesh, and with it ransomed the dove. After Buddha had attained to perfect wisdom, and in travelling about with his disciples arrived at this spot, he informed them that this was the place where he ransomed the dove with a piece of his own flesh. In this way the people of the country became aware of the fact, and on the spot reared a tope, adorned with layers of gold and silver plates.

[Footnote 1: Sakra is a common name for the Brahmanic Indra, adopted by Buddhism into the circle of its own great adherents;—it has been said, "because of his popularity." He is now the representative of the secular power, the valiant protector of the Buddhist body, but is looked upon as inferior to Sakyamuni, and every Buddhist saint.]

CHAPTER X

Gandhara—Legends of Buddha

The travellers, going downwards from this towards the east, in five days came to the country of Gandhara, the place where Dharma-vivardhana, the son of Asoka, [1] ruled. When Buddha was a Bodhisattva, he gave his eyes also for another man here; and at the spot they have also reared a large tope, adorned with layers of gold and silver plates. The people of the country were mostly students of the hinayana.

[Footnote 1: Asoka is here mentioned for the first time—the Constantine of the Buddhist society, and famous for the number of viharas and topes which he erected. He was the grandson of Chandragupta, a rude adventurer, who at one time was a refugee in the camp of Alexander the Great; and within about twenty years afterwards drove the Greeks out of India, having defeated Seleucus, the Greek ruler of the Indus provinces. His grandson was converted to Buddhism by the bold and patient demeanor of an Arhat whom he had ordered to be buried alive, and became a most zealous supporter of the new faith.]

CHAPTER XI

Takshasila—Legends—The Four Great Topes

Seven days' journey from this to the east brought the travellers to the kingdom of Takshasila, which means "the severed head" in the language of China. Here, when Buddha was a Bodhisattva, he gave away his head to a man; and from this circumstance the kingdom got its name.

Going on further for two days to the east, they came to the place where the Bodhisattva threw down his body to feed a starving tigress. In these two places also large topes have been built, both adorned with layers of all the precious substances. The kings, ministers, and peoples of the kingdoms around vie with one another in making offerings at them. The trains of those who come to scatter flowers and light lamps at them never cease. The nations of those quarters call those and the other two mentioned before "the four great topes."

CHAPTER XII

Buddha's Alms-bowl—Death of Hwuy-king

Going southwards from Gandhara, the travellers in four days arrived at the kingdom of Purushapura. [1] Formerly, when Buddha was travelling in this country with his disciples, he said to Ananda, [2] "After my pari-nirvana, [3] there will be a king named Kanishka, who shall on this spot build a tope."

This Kanishka was afterwards born into the world; and once, when he had gone forth to look about him, Sakra, Ruler of Devas, wishing to excite the idea in his mind, assumed the appearance of a little herd-boy, and was making a tope right in the way of the king, who asked what sort of a thing he was making. The boy said, "I am making a tope for Buddha." The king said, "Very good;" and immediately, right over the boy's tope, he proceeded to rear another, which was more than four hundred cubits high, and adorned with layers of all the precious substances. Of all the topes and temples which the travellers saw in their journeyings, there was not one comparable to this in solemn beauty and majestic grandeur. There is a current saying that this is the finest tope in Jambudvipa [4]. When the king's tope was completed, the little tope of the boy came out from its side on the south, rather more than three cubits in height.

Buddha's alms-bowl is in this country. Formerly, a king of Yueeh-she raised a large force and invaded this country, wishing to carry the bowl away. Having subdued the kingdom, as he and his captains were sincere believers in the Law of Buddha, and wished to carry off the bowl, they proceeded to present their offerings on a great scale. When they had done so to the Three Precious Ones, he made a large elephant be grandly caparisoned, and placed the bowl upon it. But the elephant knelt down on the ground, and was unable to go forward. Again he caused a four-wheeled wagon to be prepared in which the bowl was put to be conveyed away. Eight elephants were then yoked to it, and dragged it with their united strength; but neither were they able to go forward. The king knew that the time for an association between himself and the bowl had not yet arrived, and was sad and deeply ashamed of himself. Forthwith he built a tope at the place and a monastery, and left a guard to watch the bowl, making all sorts of contributions.

There may be there more than seven hundred monks. When it is near mid-day, they bring out the bowl, and, along with the common people, make their various offerings to it, after which they take their mid-day meal. In the evening, at the time of incense, they bring the bowl out again. It may contain rather more than two pecks, and is of various colors, black predominating, with the seams that show its fourfold composition distinctly marked. Its thickness is about the fifth of an inch, and it has a bright and glossy lustre. When poor people throw into it a few flowers, it becomes immediately full, while some very rich people, wishing to make offering of many flowers, might not stop till they had thrown in hundreds, thousands, and myriads of bushels, and yet would not be able to fill it.[5]

Pao-yun and Sang-king here merely made their offerings to the alms-bowl, and then resolved to go back. Hwuy-king, Hwuy-tah, and Tao-ching had gone on before the rest to Nagara, to make their offerings at the places of Buddha's shadow, tooth, and the flat-bone of his skull. There Hwuy-king fell ill, and Tao-ching remained to look after him, while Hwuy-tah came alone to Purushapura, and saw the others, and then he with Pao-yun and Sang-king took their way back to the land of Ts'in. Hwuy-king came to his end in the monastery of Buddha's alms-bowl, and on this Fa-hien went forward alone towards the place of the flat-bone of Buddha's skull.[6]

[Footnote 1: The modern Peshawur.]

[Footnote 2: A first cousin of Sakyamuni, and born at the moment when he attained to Buddhaship. Under Buddha's teaching, Ananda became an Arhat, and is famous for his strong and accurate memory; and he played an important part at the first council for the formation of the Buddhist canon. The friendship between Sakyamuni and Ananda was very close and tender; and it is impossible to read much of what the dying Buddha said to him and of him, as related in the Mahapari-nirvana Sutra, without being moved almost to tears. Ananda is to reappear on earth as Buddha in another Kalpa.]

[Footnote 3: On his attaining to nirvana, Sakyamuni became the Buddha, and had no longer to mourn his being within the circle of transmigration, and could rejoice in an absolute freedom from passion, and a perfect purity. Still he continued to live on for forty-five years, till he attained to pari-nirvana, and had done with all the life of sense and society, and had no more exercise of thought. He died; but whether he absolutely and entirely ceased to be, in any sense of the word being, it would be difficult to say. Probably he himself would not and could not have spoken definitely on the point. So far as our use of language is concerned, apart from any assured faith in and hope of immortality, his pari-nirvana was his death.]

[Footnote 4: Jambudvipa is one of the four great continents of the universe, representing the inhabited world as fancied by the Buddhists, and so-called because it resembles in shape the leaves of the jambu tree.]

[Footnote 5: Compare the narrative in Luke's Gospel, xxi. 1-4.]

[Footnote 6: This story of Hwuy-king's death differs from the account given in chapter xiv.—EDITOR.]

CHAPTER XIII

Festival of Buddha's Skull-bone

Going west for sixteen yojanas, [1] he came to the city He-lo [2] in the borders of the country of Nagara, where there is the flat-bone of Buddha's skull, deposited in a vihara [3] adorned all over with gold-leaf and the seven sacred substances. The king of the country, revering and honoring the bone, and anxious lest it should be stolen away, has selected eight individuals, representing the great families in the kingdom, and committed to each a seal, with which he should seal its shrine and guard the relic. At early dawn these eight men come, and after each has inspected his seal, they open the door. This done, they wash their hands with scented water and bring out the bone, which they place outside the vihara, on a lofty platform, where it is supported on a round pedestal of the seven precious substances, and covered with a bell of lapis lazuli, both adorned with rows of pearls. Its color is of a yellowish white, and it forms an imperfect circle twelve inches round, curving upwards to the centre. Every day, after it has been brought forth, the keepers of the vihara ascend a high gallery, where they beat great drums, blow conches, and clash their copper cymbals. When the king hears them, he goes to the vihara, and makes his offerings of flowers and incense. When he has done this, he and his attendants in order, one after another, raise the bone, place it for a moment on the top of their heads, and then depart, going out by the door on the west as they had entered by that on the east. The king every morning makes his offerings and performs his worship, and afterwards gives audience on the business of his government. The chiefs of the Vaisyas [4] also make their offerings before they attend to their family affairs. Every day it is so, and there is no remissness in the observance of the custom. When all of the offerings are over, they replace the bone in the vihara, where there is a vimoksha tope, of the seven precious substances, and rather more than five cubits high, sometimes open, sometimes shut, to contain it. In front of the door of the vihara, there are parties who every morning sell flowers and incense, and those who wish to make offerings buy some of all kinds. The kings of various countries are also constantly sending messengers with offerings. The vihara stands in a square of thirty paces, and though heaven should shake and earth be rent, this place would not move.

Going on, north from this, for a yojana, Fa-hien arrived at the capital of Nagara, the place where the Bodhisattva once purchased with money five stalks of flowers, as an offering to the Dipankara Buddha. In the midst of the city there is also the tope of Buddha's tooth, where offerings are made in the same way as to the flat-bone of his skull.

A yojana to the northeast of the city brought him to the mouth of a valley, where there is Buddha's pewter staff; and a vihara also has been built at which offerings are made. The staff is made of Gosirsha Chandana, and is quite sixteen or seventeen cubits long. It is contained in a wooden tube, and though a hundred or a thousand men were to try to lift it, they could not move it.

Entering the mouth of the valley, and going west, he found Buddha's Sanghali, [5] where also there is reared a vihara, and offerings are made. It is a custom of the country when there is a great drought, for the people to collect in crowds, bring out the robe, pay worship to it, and make offerings, on which there is immediately a great rain from the sky.

South of the city, half a yojana, there is a rock-cavern, in a great hill fronting the southwest; and here it was that Buddha left his shadow. Looking at it from a distance of more than ten paces, you seem to see Buddha's real form, with his complexion of gold, and his characteristic marks in their nicety, clearly and brightly displayed. The nearer you approach, however, the fainter it becomes, as if it were only in your fancy. When the kings from the regions all around have sent skilful artists to take a copy, none of them have been able to do so. Among the people of the country there is a saying current that "the thousand Buddhas must all leave their shadows here."

Rather more than four hundred paces west from the shadow, when Buddha was at the spot, he shaved off his hair and clipped his nails, and proceeded, along with his disciples, to build a tope seventy or eighty cubits high, to be a model for all future topes; and it is still existing. By the side of it there is a monastery, with more than seven hundred monks in it. At this place there are as many as a thousand topes of Arhans and Pratyeka Buddhas.

[Footnote 1: Now in India, Fa-hien used the Indian measure of distance; but it is not possible to determine exactly what its length then was. The estimates of it are very different, and vary from four and a half or five miles to seven, and sometimes more.]

[Footnote 2: The present Hidda, west of Peshawur, and five miles south of Jellalabad.]

[Footnote 3: "The vihara," says Hardy, "is the residence of a recluse or priest;" and so Davids—"the clean little hut where the mendicant lives."]

[Footnote 4: The Vaisyas, or the bourgeois caste of Hindu society, are described here as "resident scholars."]

[Footnote 5: Or Sanghati, the double or composite robe, part of a monk's attire, reaching from the shoulders to the knees, and fastened round the waist.]

CHAPTER XIV

Crossing the Indus to the East

Having stayed there till the third month of winter, Fa-hien and the two others, proceeding southwards, crossed the Little Snowy mountains. On them the snow lies accumulated both winter and summer. On the north side of the mountains, in the shade, they suddenly encountered a cold wind which made them shiver and become unable to speak. Hwuy-king could not go any farther. A white froth came from his mouth, and he said to Fa-hien, "I cannot live any longer. Do you immediately go away, that we do not all die here"; and with these words he died. Fa-hien stroked the corpse, and cried out piteously, "Our original plan has failed; it is fate. What can we do?" He then again exerted himself, and they succeeded in crossing to the south of the range, and arrived in the kingdom of Lo-e, [1] where there were nearly three thousand monks, students of both the mahayana and hinayana. Here they stayed for the summer retreat, [2] and when that was over, they went on to the south, and ten days' journey brought them to the kingdom of Poh-na, where there are also more than three thousand monks, all students of the hinayana. Proceeding from this place for three days, they again crossed the Indus, where the country on each side was low and level.

[Footnote 1: Lo-e, or Rohi, or Afghanistan; only a portion of it can be intended.]

[Footnote 2: We are now therefore in A.D. 404.]

CHAPTER XV

Sympathy of Monks with the Pilgrims

After they had crossed the river, there was a country named Pe-t'oo, where Buddhism was very flourishing, and the monks studied both the mahayana and hinayana. When they saw their fellow-disciples from Ts'in passing along, they were moved with great pity and sympathy, and expressed themselves thus: "How is it that these men from a border-land should have learned to become monks, and come for the sake of our doctrines from such a distance in search of the Law of Buddha?" They supplied them with what they needed, and treated them in accordance with the rules of the Law.

CHAPTER XVI

Condition and Customs of Central India

From this place they travelled southeast, passing by a succession of very many monasteries, with a multitude of monks, who might be counted by myriads. After passing all these places, they came to a country named Ma-t'aou-lo. They still followed the course of the P'oo-na river, on the banks of which, left and right, there were twenty monasteries, which might contain three thousand monks; and here the Law of Buddha was still more flourishing. Everywhere, from the Sandy Desert, in all the countries of India, the kings had been firm believers in that Law. When they make their offerings to a community of monks, they take off their royal caps, and along with their relatives and ministers, supply them with food with their own hands. That done, the king has a carpet spread for himself on the ground, and sits down on it in front of the chairman;—they dare not presume to sit on couches in front of the community. The laws and ways, according to which the kings presented their offerings when Buddha was in the world, have been handed down to the present day.

All south from this is named the Middle Kingdom. In it the cold and heat are finely tempered, and there is neither hoarfrost nor snow. The people are numerous and happy; they have not to register their households, or attend to any magistrates and their rules; only those who cultivate the royal land have to pay a portion of the gain from it. If they want to go they go; if they want to stay on, they stay. The king governs without decapitation or other corporal punishments. Criminals are simply fined, lightly or heavily, according to the circumstances of each case. Even in cases of repeated attempts at wicked rebellion, they only have their right hands cut off. The king's body-guards and attendants all have salaries. Throughout the whole country the people do not kill any living creature, nor drink intoxicating liquor, nor eat onions or garlic. The only exception is that of the Chandalas. That is the name for those who are held to be wicked men, and live apart from others. When they enter the gate of a city or a market-place, they strike a piece of wood to make themselves known, so that men know and avoid them, and do not come into contact with them. In that country they do not keep pigs and fowls, and do not sell live cattle; in the markets there are no butchers' shops and no dealers in intoxicating drink. In buying and selling commodities they use cowries. Only the Chandalas are fishermen and hunters, and sell flesh meat.

After Buddha attained to pari-nirvana the kings of the various countries and the heads of the Vaisyas built viharas for the priests, and endowed them with fields, houses, gardens, and orchards, along with the resident populations and their cattle, the grants being engraved on plates of metal, so that afterwards they were handed down from king to king, without any one daring to annul them, and they remain even to the present time.

The regular business of the monks is to perform acts of meritorious virtue, and to recite their Sutras and sit wrapped in meditation. When stranger monks arrive at any monastery, the old residents meet and receive them, carry for them their clothes and alms-bowl, give them water to wash their feet, oil with which to anoint them, and the liquid food permitted out of the regular hours. [1] When the stranger has enjoyed a very brief rest, they further ask the number of years that he has been a monk, after which he receives a sleeping apartment with its appurtenances, according to his regular order, and everything is done for him which the rules prescribe.

Where a community of monks resides, they erect topes to Sariputtra, [2] to Maha-maudgalyayana, [3] and to Ananda, and also topes in honor of the Abhidharma, [4] the Vinaya, [4] and the Sutras. [4] A month after the annual season of rest, the families which are looking out for blessing stimulate one another to make offerings to the monks, and send round to them the liquid food which may be taken out of the ordinary hours. All the monks come together in a great assembly, and preach the Law; after which offerings are presented at the tope of Sariputtra, with all kinds of flowers and incense. All through the night lamps are kept burning, and skilful musicians are employed to perform.

When Sariputtra was a great Brahman, he went to Buddha, and begged to be permitted to quit his family and become a monk. The great Mugalan and the great Kas'yapa also did the same. The bhikshunis [5] for the most part make their offerings at the tope of Ananda, because it was he who requested the World-honored one to allow females to quit their families and become nuns. The Sramaneras [6] mostly make their offerings to Rahula. [7] The professors of the Abhidharma make their offerings to it; those of the Vinaya to it. Every year there is one such offering, and each class has its own day for it. Students of the mahayana present offerings to the Prajna-paramita, to Manjus'ri, and to Kwan-she-yin. When the monks have done receiving their annual tribute from the harvests, the Heads of the Vaisyas and all the Brahmans bring clothes and such other articles as the monks require for use, and distribute among them. The monks, having received them, also proceed to give portions to one another. From the nirvana of Buddha, the forms of ceremony, laws, and rules, practised by the sacred communities, have been handed down from one generation to another without interruption.

From the place where the travellers crossed the Indus to South India, and on to the Southern Sea, a distance of forty or fifty thousand li, all is level plain. There are no large hills with streams among them; there are simply the waters of the rivers.

[Footnote 1: No monk can eat solid food except between sunrise and noon, and total abstinence from intoxicating drinks is obligatory. Food eaten at any other part of the day is called vikala, and forbidden; but a weary traveller might receive unseasonable refreshment, consisting of honey, butter, treacle, and sesamum oil.]

[Footnote 2: Sariputtra was one of the principal disciples of Buddha, and indeed the most learned and ingenious of them all.]

[Footnote 3: Mugalan, the Singhalese name of this disciple, is more pronounceable. He also was one of the principal disciples, called Buddha's "left-hand attendant." He was distinguished for his power of vision, and his magic powers.]

[Footnote 4: The different parts of the tripitaka.]

[Footnote 5: The bhikshunis are the female monks or nuns, subject to the same rules as the bhikshus, and also to special ordinances of restraint.]

[Footnote 6: The Sramaneras are the novices, male or female, who have vowed to observe the Shikshapada, or ten commandments.]

[Footnote 7: The eldest son of Sakyamuni by Yasodhara. Converted to Buddhism, he followed his father as an attendant; and after Buddha's death became the founder of a philosophical realistic school (vaibhashika). He is now revered as the patron saint of all novices, and is to be reborn as the eldest son of every future Buddha.]

CHAPTER XVII

Legend of the Trayastrimsas Heaven

From this they proceeded southeast for eighteen yojanas, and found themselves in a kingdom called Sankas'ya, at the place where Buddha came down, after ascending to the Trayastrims'as heaven [1], and there preaching for three months his Law for the benefit of his mother [2]. Buddha had gone up to this heaven by his supernatural power, without letting his disciples know; but seven days before the completion of the three months he laid aside his invisibility, and Anuruddha [3], with his heavenly eyes, saw the World-honored one, and immediately said to the honored one, the great Mugalan, "Do you go and salute the World-honored one," Mugalan forthwith went, and with head and face did homage at Buddha's feet. They then saluted and questioned each other, and when this was over, Buddha said to Mugalan, "Seven days after this I will go down to Jambudvipa"; and thereupon Mugalan returned. At this time the great kings of eight countries with their ministers and people, not having seen Buddha for a long time, were all thirstily looking up for him, and had collected in clouds in this kingdom to wait for the World-honored one.

Then the bhikshuni Utpala thought in her heart, "To-day the kings, with their ministers and people, will all be meeting and welcoming Buddha. I am but a woman; how shall I succeed in being the first to see him?" Buddha immediately, by his spirit-like power, changed her into the appearance of a holy Chakravartti king, and she was the foremost of all in doing reverence to him.

As Buddha descended from his position aloft in the Trayastrims'as heaven, when he was coming down, there were made to appear three flights of precious steps. Buddha was on the middle flight, the steps of which were composed of the seven precious substances. The king of Brahma-loka [4] also made a flight of silver steps appear on the right side, where he was seen attending with a white chowry in his hand. Sakra, Ruler of Devas, made a flight of steps of purple gold on the left side, where he was seen attending and holding an umbrella of the seven precious substances. An innumerable multitude of the devas followed Buddha in his descent. When he was come down, the three flights all disappeared in the ground, excepting seven steps, which continued to be visible. Afterwards king As'oka, wishing to know where their ends rested, sent men to dig and see. They went down to the yellow springs without reaching the bottom of the steps, and from this the king received an increase to his reverence and faith, and built a vihara over the steps, with a standing image, sixteen cubits in height, right over the middle flight. Behind the vihara he erected a stone pillar, about fifty cubits high, with a lion on the top of it. [5] Let into the pillar, on each of its four sides, there is an image of Buddha, inside and out shining and transparent, and pure as it were of lapis lazuli. Some teachers of another doctrine once disputed with the S'ramanas about the right to this as a place of residence, and the latter were having the worst of the argument, when they took an oath on both sides on the condition that, if the place did indeed belong to the S'ramanas, there should be some marvellous attestation of it. When these words had been spoken, the lion on the top gave a great roar, thus giving the proof; on which their opponents were frightened, bowed to the decision, and withdrew.

Through Buddha having for three months partaken of the food of heaven, his body emitted a heavenly fragrance, unlike that of an ordinary man. He went immediately and bathed; and afterwards, at the spot where he did so, a bathing-house was built, which is still existing. At the place where the bhikshuni Utpala was the first to do reverence to Buddha, a tope has now been built.

At the places where Buddha, when he was in the world, cut his hair and nails, topes are erected; and where the three Buddhas [6] that preceded S'akyamuni Buddha and he himself sat; where they walked, and where images of their persons were made. At all these places topes were made, and are still existing. At the place where S'akra, Ruler of the Devas, and the king of the Brahma-loka followed Buddha down from the Trayastrimsas heaven they have also raised a tope.

At this place the monks and nuns may be a thousand, who all receive their food from the common store, and pursue their studies, some of the mahayana and some of the hinayana. Where they live, there is a white-eared dragon, which acts the part of danapati to the community of these monks, causing abundant harvests in the country, and the enriching rains to come in season, without the occurrence of any calamities, so that the monks enjoy their repose and ease. In gratitude for its kindness, they have made for it a dragon-house, with a carpet for it to sit on, and appointed for it a diet of blessing, which they present for its nourishment. Every day they set apart three of their number to go to its house, and eat there. Whenever the summer retreat is ended, the dragon straightway changes its form, and appears as a small snake, with white spots at the side of its ears. As soon as the monks recognize it, they fill a copper vessel with cream, into which they put the creature, and then carry it round from the one who has the highest seat at their tables to him who has the lowest, when it appears as if saluting them. When it has been taken round, immediately it disappears; and every year it thus comes forth once. The country is very productive, and the people are prosperous, and happy beyond comparison. When people of other countries come to it, they are exceedingly attentive to them all, and supply them with what they need.

Fifty yojanas northwest from the monastery there is another, called "The Great Heap." Great Heap was the name of a wicked demon, who was converted by Buddha, and men subsequently at this place reared a vihara. When it was being made over to an Arhat by pouring water on his hands, some drops fell on the ground. They are still on the spot, and however they may be brushed away and removed, they continue to be visible, and cannot be made to disappear.

At this place there is also a tope to Buddha, where a good spirit constantly keeps all about it swept and watered, without any labor of man being required. A king of corrupt views once said, "Since you are able to do this, I will lead a multitude of troops and reside there till the dirt and filth has increased and accumulated, and see whether you can cleanse it away or not." The spirit thereupon raised a great wind, which blew the filth away, and made the place pure.

At this place there are many small topes, at which a man may keep counting a whole day without being able to know their exact number. If he be firmly bent on knowing it, he will place a man by the side of each tope. When this is done, proceeding to count the number of the men, whether they be many or few, he will not get to know the number. [7]

There is a monastery, containing perhaps six hundred or seven hundred monks, in which there is a place where a Pratyeka Buddha used to take his food. The nirvana ground where he was burned after death is as large as a carriage wheel; and while grass grows all around, on this spot there is none. The ground also where he dried his clothes produces no grass, but the impression of them, where they lay on it, continues to the present day.

[Footnote 1: The heaven of Indra or Sakya, meaning "the heaven of thirty-three classes," a name which has been explained both historically and mythologically. "The description of it," says Eitel, "tallies in all respects with the Svarga of Brahmanic mythology. It is situated between the four peaks of the Meru, and consists of thirty-two cities of devas, eight on each of the four corners of the mountain. Indra's capital of Bellevue is in the centre. There he is enthroned, with a thousand heads and a thousand eyes, and four arms grasping the vajra, with his wife and 119,000 concubines. There he receives the monthly reports of the four Maharajas, concerning the progress of good and evil in the world," *etc., etc.*]

[Footnote 2: Buddha's mother, Maya and Maha-maya, died seven days after his birth.]

[Footnote 3: Anuruddha was a first cousin of Sakyamuni, being the son of his uncle Amritodana. He is often mentioned in the account we have of Buddha's last moments. His special gift was the "heavenly eye," the first of the six "supernatural talents," the faculty of comprehending in one instantaneous view, or by intuition, all beings in all worlds.]

[Footnote 4: This was Brahma, the first person of the Brahmanical Trimurti, adopted by Buddhism, but placed in an inferior position, and surpassed by every Buddhist saint who attains to bodhi.]

[Footnote 5: A note of Mr. Beal says on this:—"General Cunningham, who visited the spot (1862), found a pillar, evidently of the age of Asoka, with a well-carved elephant on the top, which, however, was minus trunk and tail. He supposes this to be the pillar seen by Fa-hien, who mistook the top of it for a lion. It is possible such a mistake may have been made, as in the account of one of the pillars at Sravasti, Fa-hien says an ox formed the capital, whilst Hsuean-chwang calls it an elephant."]

[Footnote 6: These three predecessors of Sakya-muni were the three Buddhas of the present or Maha-bhadra Kalpa, of which he was the fourth, and Maitreya is to be the fifth and last. They were: (i) Kra-kuchanda, "he who readily solves all doubts"; a scion of the Kasyapa family. Human life reached in his time forty thousand years, and so many persons were converted by him. (2) Kanakamuni, "body radiant with the color of pure gold"; of the same family. Human life reached in his time thirty thousand years, and so many persons were converted by him. (3) Kasyapa, "swallower of light." Human life reached in his time twenty thousand years, and so many persons were converted by him.]

[Footnote 7: This would seem to be absurd; but the writer evidently intended to convey the idea that there was something mysterious about the number of the topes.]

CHAPTER XVIII

Buddha's Subjects of Discourse

Fa-Hien stayed at the Dragon vihara till after the summer retreat, [1] and then, travelling to the southeast for seven yojanas, he arrived at the city of Kanyakubja, lying along the Ganges. There are two monasteries in it, the inmates of which are students of the hinayana. At a distance from the city of six or seven li, on the west, on the northern bank of the Ganges, is a place where Buddha preached the Law to his disciples. It has been handed down that his subjects of discourse were such as "The bitterness and vanity of life as impermanent and uncertain," and that "The body is as a bubble or foam on the water." At this spot a tope was erected, and still exists.

Having crossed the Ganges, and gone south for three yojanas, the travellers arrived at a village named A-le, containing places where Buddha preached the Law, where he sat, and where he walked, at all of which topes have been built.

[Footnote 1: This was, probably, in A.D. 405.]

CHAPTER XIX

Legend of Buddha's Danta-kashtha

Going on from this to the southeast for three yojanas, they came to the great kingdom of Sha-che. As you go out of the city of Sha-che by the southern gate, on the east of the road is the place where Buddha, after he had chewed his willow branch, stuck it in the ground, when it forthwith grew up seven cubits, at which height it remained, neither increasing nor diminishing. The Brahmans, with their contrary doctrines, became angry and jealous. Sometimes they cut the tree down, sometimes they plucked it up, and cast it to a distance, but it grew again on the same spot as at first. Here also is the place where the four Buddhas walked and sat, and at which a tope was built that is still existing.

CHAPTER XX

The Jetavana Vihara—Legends of Buddha

Going on from this to the south, for eight yojanas, the travellers came to the city of Sravasti in the kingdom of Kosala, in which the inhabitants were few and far between, amounting in all only to a few more than two hundred families; the city where king Prasenajit ruled, and the place of the old vihara of Maha-prajapati; [1] of the well and walls of the house of the Vaisya head Sudatta; [2] and where the Angulimalya [3] became an Arhat, and his body was afterwards burned on his attaining to pari-nirvana. At all these places topes were subsequently erected, which are still existing in the city. The Brahmans, with their contrary doctrine, became full of hatred and envy in their hearts, and wished to destroy them, but there came from the heavens such a storm of crashing thunder and flashing lightning that they were not able in the end to effect their purpose.

As you go out from the city by the south gate, and one thousand two hundred paces from it, the Vais'ya head Sudatta built a vihara, facing the south; and when the door was open, on each side of it there was a stone pillar, with the figure of a wheel on the top of that on the left, and the figure of an ox on the top of that on the right. On the left and right of the building the ponds of water clear and pure, the thickets of trees always luxuriant, and the numerous flowers of various hues, constituted a lovely scene, the whole forming what is called the Jetavana vihara.

When Buddha went up to the Trayastrimsas heaven, and preached the Law for the benefit of his mother, after he had been absent for ninety days, Prasenajit, longing to see him, caused an image of him to be carved in Gosirsha Chandana wood, and put in the place where he usually sat. When Buddha, on his return entered the vihara, this image immediately left its place, and came forth to meet him. Buddha said to it, "Return to your seat. After I have attained to pari-nirvana, you will serve as a pattern to the four classes of my disciples," [4] and on this the image returned to its seat. This was the very first of all the images of Buddha, and that which men subsequently copied. Buddha then removed, and dwelt in a small vihara on the south side of the other, a different place from that containing the image, and twenty paces distant from it.

The Jetavana vihara was originally of seven stories. The kings and people of the countries around vied with one another in their offerings, hanging up about it silken streamers and canopies, scattering flowers, burning incense, and lighting lamps, so as to make the night as bright as the day. This they did day after day without ceasing. It happened that a rat, carrying in its mouth the wick of a lamp, set one of the streamers or canopies on fire, which caught the vihara, and the seven stories were all consumed. The kings, with their officers and people, were all very sad and distressed, supposing that the sandalwood image had been burned; but lo! after four or five days, when the door of a small vihara on the east was opened, there was immediately seen the original image. They were all greatly rejoiced, and cooperated in restoring the vihara. When they had succeeded in completing two stories, they removed the image back to its former place.

When Fa-hien and Tao-ching first arrived at the Jetavana monastery, and thought how the World-honored one had formerly resided there for twenty-five years, painful reflections arose in their minds. Born in a border-land, along with their like-minded friends, they had travelled through so many kingdoms; some of those friends had returned to their own land, and some had died, proving the impermanence and uncertainty of life; and today they saw the place where Buddha had lived now unoccupied by him. They were melancholy through their pain of heart, and the crowd of monks came out, and asked them from what kingdom they were come. "We are come," they replied, "from the land of Han." "Strange," said the monks with a sigh, "that men of a border country should be able to come here in search of our Law!" Then they said to one another, "During all the time that we, preceptors and monks, have succeeded to one another, we have never seen men of Han, followers of our system, arrive here."

Four li to the northwest of the vihara there is a grove called "The Getting of Eyes." Formerly there were five hundred blind men, who lived here in order that they might be near the vihara. Buddha preached his Law to them, and they all got their eyesight. Full of joy, they stuck their staves in the earth, and with their heads and faces on the ground, did reverence. The staves immediately began to grow, and they grew to be great. People made much of them, and no one dared to cut them down, so that they came to form a grove. It was in this way that it got its name, and most of the Jetavana monks, after they had taken their mid-day meal, went to the grove, and sat there in meditation.

Six or seven li northeast from the Jetavana, mother Vaisakha built another vihara, to which she invited Buddha and his monks, and which is still existing.

To each of the great residences for the monks at the Jetavana vihara there were two gates, one facing the east and the other facing the north. The park containing the whole was the space of ground which the Vaisaya head, Sudatta, purchased by covering it with gold coins. The vihara was exactly in the centre. Here Buddha lived for a longer time than at any other place, preaching his Law and converting men. At the places where he walked and sat they also subsequently reared topes, each having its particular name; and here was the place where Sundari [5] murdered a person and then falsely charged Buddha with the crime. Outside the east gate of the Jetavana, at a distance of seventy paces to the north, on the west of the road, Buddha held a discussion with the advocates of the ninety-six schemes of erroneous doctrine, when the king and his great officers, the householders, and people were all assembled in crowds to hear it. Then a woman belonging to one of the erroneous systems, by name Chanchamana, prompted by the envious hatred in her heart, and having put on extra clothes in front of her person, so as to give her the appearance of being with child, falsely accused Buddha before all the assembly of having acted unlawfully towards her. On this, Sakra, Ruler of Devas, changed himself and some devas into white mice, which bit through the strings about her waist; and when this was done, the extra clothes which she wore dropped down on the ground. The earth at the same time was rent, and she went down alive into hell. This also is the place where Devadatta, trying with empoisoned claws to injure Buddha, went down alive into hell. Men subsequently set up marks to distinguish where both these events took place.

Further, at the place where the discussion took place, they reared a vihara rather more than sixty cubits high, having in it an image of Buddha in a sitting posture. On the east of the road there was a devalaya [6] of one of the contrary systems, called "The Shadow Covered," right opposite the vihara on the place of discussion, with only the road between them, and also rather more than sixty cubits high. The reason why it was called "The Shadow Covered" was this: When the sun was in the west, the shadow of the vihara of the World-honored one fell on the devalaya of a contrary system; but when the sun was in the east, the shadow of that devalaya was diverted to the north, and never fell on the vihara of Buddha. The malbelievers regularly employed men to watch their devalaya, to sweep and water all about it, to burn incense, light the lamps, and present offerings; but in the morning the lamps were found to have been suddenly removed, and in the vihara of Buddha. The Brahmans were indignant, and said, "Those Sramanas take our lamps and use them for their own service of Buddha, but we will not stop our service for you!" [7] On that night the Brahmans themselves kept watch, when they saw the deva spirits which they served take the lamps and go three times round the vihara of Buddha and present offerings. After this administration to Buddha they suddenly disappeared. The Brahmans thereupon knowing how great was the spiritual power of Buddha, forthwith left their families, and became monks. It has been handed down, that, near the time when these things occurred, around the Jetavana vihara there were ninety-eight monasteries, in all of which there were monks residing, excepting only in one place which was vacant. In this Middle Kingdom there are ninety-six sorts of views, erroneous and different from our system, all of which recognize this world and the future world and the connection between them. Each has its multitude of followers, and they all beg their food: only they do not carry the alms-bowl. They also, moreover, seek to acquire the blessing of good deeds on unfrequented ways, setting up on the roadside houses of charity, where rooms, couches, beds, and food and drink are supplied to travellers, and also to monks, coming and going as guests, the only difference being in the time for which those parties remain.

There are also companies of the followers of Devadatta still existing. They regularly make offerings to the three previous Buddhas, but not to Sakyamuni Buddha.

Four li southeast from the city of Sravasti, a tope has been erected at the place where the World-honored one encountered king Virudhaha, when he wished to attack the kingdom of Shay-e, and took his stand before him at the side of the road.

[Footnote 1: Explained by "Path of Love," and "Lord of Life." Prajapati was aunt and nurse of Sakyamuni, the first woman admitted to the monkhood, and the first superior of the first Buddhistic convent. She is yet to become a Buddha.]

[Footnote 2: Sudatta, meaning "almsgiver," was the original name of Anathapindika, a wealthy householder, or Vaisya head, of Sravasti, famous for his liberality. Of his old house, only the well and walls remained at the time of Fa-hien's visit to Sravasti.]

[Footnote 3: The Angulimalya were a sect or set of Sivaitic fanatics, who made assassination a religious act. The one of them here mentioned had joined them by the force of circumstances. Being converted by Buddha, he became a monk.]

[Footnote 4: Arya, meaning "honorable," "venerable," is a title given only to those who have mastered the four spiritual truths:—(i) that "misery" is a necessary condition of all sentient existence; this is duhka: (ii) that the "accumulation" of misery is caused by the passions; this is samudaya: (iii) that the "extinction" of passion is possible; this is nirodha: and (iv) that the "path" leads to the extinction of passion; which is marga. According to their attainment of these truths, the Aryas, or followers of Buddha, are distinguished into four classes—Srotapannas, Sakridagamins, Anagamins, and Arhats.]

[Footnote 5: Hsuean-chwang does not give the name of this murderer; see in Julien's "Vie et Voyages de Hiouen-thsang "—"a heretical Brahman killed a woman and calumniated Buddha." See also the fuller account in Beal's "Records of Western Countries," where the murder is committed by several Brahmacharins. In this passage Beal makes Sundari to be the name of the murdered person. But the text cannot be so construed.]

[Footnote 6: A devalaya is a place in which a deva is worshipped—a general name for all Brahmanical temples.]

[Footnote 7: Their speech was somewhat unconnected, but natural enough in the circumstances. Compare the whole account with the narrative in 1 Samuel v. about the Ark and Dagon, that "twice-battered god of Palestine."]

CHAPTER XXI

The Three Predecessors of Sakyamuni

Fifty li to the west of the city brings the traveller to a town named Too-wei, the birthplace of Kasyapa Buddha. At the place where he and his father met, and at that where he attained to pari-nirvana, topes were erected. Over the entire relic of the whole body of him, the Kasyapa Tathagata, a great tope was also erected.

Going on southeast from the city of Sravasti for twelve yojanas, the travellers came to a town named Na-pei-kea, the birthplace of Krakuchanda Buddha. At the place where he and his father met, and at that where he attained to pari-nirvana, topes were erected. Going north from here less than a yojana, they came to a town which had been the birthplace of Kanakamuni Buddha. At the place where he and his father met, and where he attained to pari-nirvana, topes were erected.

CHAPTER XXII

Legends of Buddha's Birth

Less than a yojana to the east from this brought them to the city of Kapilavastu; but in it there was neither king nor people. All was mound and desolation. Of inhabitants there were only some monks and a score or two of families of the common people. At the spot where stood the old palace of king Suddhodana there have been made images of his eldest son and his mother; and at the places where that son appeared mounted on a white elephant when he entered his mother's womb, and where he turned his carriage round on seeing the sick man after he had gone out of the city by the eastern gate, topes have been erected. The places were also pointed out where the rishi A-e inspected the marks of Buddhaship on the body of the heir-apparent when an infant; where, when he was in company with Nanda and others, on the elephant being struck down and drawn on one side, he tossed it away; [1] where he shot an arrow to the southeast, and it went a distance of thirty li, then entering the ground and making a spring to come forth, which men subsequently fashioned into a well from which travellers might drink; where, after he had attained to Wisdom, Buddha returned and saw the king, his father; where five hundred Sakyas quitted their families and did reverence to Upali [2] while the earth shook and moved in six different ways; where Buddha preached his Law to the devas, and the four deva kings and others kept the four doors of the hall, so that even the king, his father, could not enter; where Buddha sat under a nyagrodha tree, which is still standing, with his face to the east, and his aunt Maha-prajapati presented him with a Sanghali; and where king Vaidurya slew the seed of Sakya, and they all in dying became Srotapannas. [3] A tope was erected at this last place, which is still existing.

Several li northeast from the city was the king's field, where the heir-apparent sat under a tree, and looked at the ploughers.

Fifty li east from the city was a garden, named Lumbini, where the queen entered the pond and bathed. Having come forth from the pond on the northern bank, after walking twenty paces, she lifted up her hand, laid hold of a branch of a tree, and, with her face to the east, gave birth to the heir-apparent. When he fell to the ground, he immediately walked seven paces. Two dragon-kings appeared and washed his body. At the place where they did so, there was immediately formed a well, and from it, as well as from the above pond, where the queen bathed, the monks even now constantly take the water, and drink it.

There are four places of regular and fixed occurrence in the history of all Buddhas: first, the place where they attained to perfect Wisdom and became Buddha; second, the place where they turned the wheel of the Law; third, the place where they preached the Law, discoursed of righteousness, and discomfited the advocates of erroneous doctrines; and fourth, the place where they came down, after going up to the Trayastrimsas heaven to preach the Law for the benefit of their mothers. Other places in connection with them became remarkable, according to the manifestations which were made at them at particular times.

The country of Kapilavastu is a great scene of empty desolation. The inhabitants are few and far between. On the roads people have to be on their guard against white elephants [4] and lions, and should not travel incautiously.

[Footnote 1: The Lichchhavis of Vaisali had sent to the young prince a very fine elephant; but when it was near Kapilavastu, Deva-datta, out of envy, killed it with a blow of his fist. Nanda (not Ananda, but a half-brother of Siddhartha), coming that way, saw the carcass lying on the road, and pulled it on one side; but the Bodhisattva, seeing it there, took it by the tail, and tossed it over seven fences and ditches, when the force of its fall made a great ditch.]

[Footnote 2: They did this, probably, to show their humility, for Upali was only a Sudra by birth, and had been a barber; so from the first did Buddhism assert its superiority to the conditions of rank and caste. Upali was distinguished by his knowledge of the rules of discipline, and praised on that account by Buddha. He was one of the three leaders of the first synod, and the principal compiler of the original Vinaya books.]

[Footnote 3: The Srotapannas are the first class of saints, who are not to be reborn in a lower sphere, but attain to nirvana after having been reborn seven times consecutively as men or devas. The Chinese editions state there were one thousand of the Sakya seed. The general account is that they were five hundred, all maidens, who refused to take their place in king Vaidurya's harem, and were in consequence taken to a pond, and had their hands and feet cut off. There Buddha came to them, had their wounds dressed, and preached to them the Law. They died in the faith, and were reborn in the region of the four Great Kings. Thence they came back and visited Buddha at Jetavana in the night, and there they obtained the reward of Srotapanna.]

[Footnote 4: Fa-hien does not say that he himself saw any of these white elephants, nor does he speak of the lions as of any particular color. We shall find by and by, in a note further on, that, to make them appear more terrible, they are spoken of as "black."]

CHAPTER XXIII

Legends of Rama and its Tope

East from Buddha's birthplace, and at a distance of five yojanas, there is a kingdom called Rama. The king of this country, having obtained one portion of the relics of Buddha's body, returned with it and built over it a tope, named the Rama tope. By the side of it there was a pool, and in the pool a dragon, which constantly kept watch over the tope, and presented offerings at it day and night. When king Asoka came forth into the world, he wished to destroy the eight topes over the relics, and to build instead of them eighty-four thousand topes. [1] After he had thrown down the seven others, he wished next to destroy this tope. But then the dragon showed itself, and took the king into its palace; when he had seen all the things provided for offerings, it said to him, "If you are able with your offerings to exceed these, you can destroy the tope, and take it all away. I will not contend with you." The king, however, knew that such appliances for offerings were not to be had anywhere in the world, and thereupon returned without carrying out his purpose.

Afterwards, the ground all about became overgrown with vegetation, and there was nobody to sprinkle and sweep about the tope; but a herd of elephants came regularly, which brought water with their trunks to water the ground, and various kinds of flowers and incense, which they presented at the tope. Once there came from one of the kingdoms a devotee to worship at the tope. When he encountered the elephants he was greatly alarmed, and screened himself among the trees; but when he saw them go through with the offerings in the most proper manner, the thought filled him with great sadness—that there should be no monastery here, the inmates of which might serve the tope, but the elephants have to do the watering and sweeping. Forthwith he gave up the great prohibitions by which he was bound, and resumed the status of a Sramanera. With his own hands he cleared away the grass and trees, put the place in good order, and made it pure and clean. By the power of his exhortations, he prevailed on the king of the country to form a residence for monks; and when that was done, he became head of the monastery. At the present day there are monks residing in it. This event is of recent occurrence; but in all the succession from that time till now, there has always been a Sramanera head of the establishment.

[Footnote 1: The bones of the human body are supposed to consist of 84,000 atoms, and hence the legend of Asoka's wish to build 84,000 topes, one over each atom of Sakyamuni's skeleton.]

CHAPTER XXIV

Where Buddha Renounced the World

East from here four yojanas, there is the place where the heir-apparent sent back Chandaka, with his white horse; and there also a tope was erected.

Four yojanas to the east from this, the travellers came to the Charcoal tope, where there is also a monastery.

Going on twelve yojanas, still to the east, they came to the city of Kusanagara, on the north of which, between two trees, on the bank of the Nairanjana river, is the place where the World-honored one, with his head to the north, attained to pan-nirvana and died. There also are the places where Subhadra, [1] the last of his converts, attained to Wisdom and became an Arhat; where in his coffin of gold they made offerings to the World-honored one for seven days, where the Vajrapani laid aside his golden club, and where the eight kings divided the relics of the burnt body: at all these places were built topes and monasteries, all of which are now existing.

In the city the inhabitants are few and far between, comprising only the families belonging to the different societies of monks.

Going from this to the southeast for twelve yojanas, they came to the place where the Lichchhavis wished to follow Buddha to the place of his pari-nirvana, and where, when he would not listen to them and they kept cleaving to him, unwilling to go away, he made to appear a large and deep ditch which they could not cross over, and gave them his alms-bowl, as a pledge of his regard, thus sending them back to their families. There a stone pillar was erected with an account of this event engraved upon it.

[Footnote 1: A Brahman of Benares, said to have been one hundred and twenty years old, who came to learn from Buddha the very night he died. Ananda would have repulsed him; but Buddha ordered him to be introduced; and then putting aside the ingenious but unimportant question which he propounded, preached to him the Law. The Brahman was converted and attained at once to Arhatship.]

CHAPTER XXV

The Kingdom of Vaisali

East from this city ten yojanas, the travellers came to the kingdom of Vaisali. North of the city so named is a large forest, having in it the double-galleried vihara where Buddha dwelt, and the tope over half the body of Ananda. Inside the city the woman Ambapali [1] built a vihara in honor of Buddha, which is now standing as it was at first. Three li south of the city, on the west of the road, is the garden which the same Ambapali presented to Buddha, in which he might reside. When Buddha was about to attain to his pari-nirvana, as he was quitting the city by the west gate, he turned round, and, beholding the city on his right, said to them, "Here I have taken my last walk." Men subsequently built a tope at this spot.

Three li northwest of the city there is a tope called, "Bows and weapons laid down." The reason why it got that name was this: The inferior wife of a king, whose country lay along the river Ganges, brought forth from her womb a ball of flesh. The superior wife, jealous of the other, said, "You have brought forth a thing of evil omen," and immediately it was put into a box of wood and thrown into the river. Farther down the stream another king was walking and looking about, when he saw the wooden box floating in the water. He had it brought to him, opened it, and found a thousand little boys, upright and complete, and each one different from the others. He took them and had them brought up. They grew tall and large, and very daring and strong, crushing all opposition in every expedition which they undertook. By and by they attacked the kingdom of their real father, who became in consequence greatly distressed and sad. His inferior wife asked what it was that made him so, and he replied, "That king has a thousand sons, daring and strong beyond compare, and he wishes with them to attack my kingdom; this is what makes me sad." The wife said, "You need not be sad and sorrowful. Only make a high gallery on the wall of the city on the east; and when the thieves come, I shall be able to make them retire." The king did as she said; and when the enemies came, she said to them from the tower, "You are my sons; why are you acting so unnaturally and rebelliously?" They replied, "Who are you that say you are our mother?" "If you do not believe me," she said, "look, all of you, towards me, and open your mouths." She then pressed her breasts with her two hands, and each sent forth five hundred jets of milk, which fell into the mouths of the thousand sons. The thieves thus knew that she was their mother, and laid down their bows and weapons. The two kings, the fathers, hereupon fell into reflection, and both got to be Pratyeka Buddhas. The tope of the two Pratyeka Buddhas is still existing.

In a subsequent age, when the World-honored one had attained to perfect Wisdom and become Buddha, he said to his disciples, "This is the place where I in a former age laid down my bow and weapons." [2] It was thus that subsequently men got to know the fact, and raised the tope on this spot, which in this way received its name. The thousand little boys were the thousand Buddhas of this Bhadra-kalpa. [3]

It was by the side of the "Weapons-laid-down" tope that Buddha, having given up the idea of living longer, said to Ananda, "In three months from this I will attain to pari-nirvana"; and king Mara [4] had so fascinated and stupefied Ananda, that he was not able to ask Buddha to remain longer in this world.

Three or four li east from this place there is a tope commemorating the following occurrence: A hundred years after the pari-nirvana of Buddha, some Bhikshus of Vaisali went wrong in the matter of the disciplinary rules in ten particulars, and appealed for their justification to what they said were the words of Buddha. Hereupon the Arhats and Bhikshus observant of the rules, to the number in all of seven hundred monks, examined afresh and collated the collection of disciplinary books [5]. Subsequently men built at this place the tope in question, which is still existing.

[Footnote 1: Ambapali, Amrapali, or Amradarika, "the guardian of the Amra (probably the mango) tree," is famous in Buddhist annals. She was a courtesan. She had been in many narakas or hells, was one hundred thousand times a female beggar, and ten thousand times a prostitute; but maintaining perfect continence during the period of Kasyana Buddha, Sakyamuni's predecessor, she had been born a devi, and finally appeared in earth under an Amra tree in Vaisali. There again she fell into her old ways, and had a son by king Bimbisara; but she was won over by Buddha to virtue and chastity, renounced the world, and attained to the state of an Arhat.]

[Footnote 2: Thus Sakyamuni had been one of the thousand little boys who floated in the box in the Ganges. How long back the former age was we cannot tell. I suppose the tope of the two fathers who became Pratyeka Buddhas had been built like the one commemorating the laying down of weapons after Buddha had told his disciples of the strange events in the past.]

[Footnote 3: Bhadra-kalpa, "the Kalpa of worthies or sages." "This," says Eitel, "is a designation for a Kalpa of stability, so-called because one thousand Buddhas appear in the course of it. Our present period is a Bhadra-kalpa, and four Buddhas have already appeared. It is to last two hundred and thirty-six millions of years, but over one hundred and fifty-one millions have already elapsed."]

[Footnote 4: "The king of demons." The name Mara is explained by "the murderer," "the destroyer of virtue," and similar appellations. "He is," says Eitel, "the personification of lust, the god of love, sin, and death, the arch-enemy of goodness, residing in the heaven Paranirmita Vasavartin on the top of the Kamadhatu. He assumes different forms, especially monstrous ones, to tempt or frighten the saints, or sends his daughters, or inspires wicked men like Devadatta or the Nirgranthas to do his work. He is often represented with 100 arms, and riding on an elephant."]

[Footnote 5: Or the Vinaya-pitaka. The meeting referred to was an important one, and is generally spoken of as the second Great Council of the Buddhist Church. The first Council was that held at Rajagriha, shortly after Buddha's death, under the presidency of Kasyapa—say about B.C. 410. The second was that spoken of here—say about B.C. 300.]

CHAPTER XXVI

Remarkable Death of Ananda

Four yojanas on from this place to the east brought the travellers to the confluence of the five rivers. When Ananda was going from Magadha to Vaisali, wishing his pari-nirvana to take place there, the devas informed king Ajatasatru [1] of it, and the king immediately pursued him, in his own grand carriage, with a body of soldiers, and had reached the river. On the other hand, the Lichchhavis of Vaisali had heard that Ananda was coming to their city, and they on their part came to meet him. In this way, they all arrived together at the river, and Ananda considered that, if he went forward, king Ajatasatru would be very angry, while, if he went back, the Lichchhavis would resent his conduct. He thereupon in the very middle of the river burnt his body in a fiery ecstasy of Samadhi [2], and his pari-nirvana was attained. He divided his body into two parts, leaving one part on each bank; so that each of the two kings got one part as a sacred relic, and took it back to his own capital, and there raised a tope over it.

[Footnote 1: He was the son of king Bimbisara, who was one of the first royal converts to Buddhism. Ajasat murdered his father, or at least wrought his death; and was at first opposed to Sakyamuni, and a favorer of Devadotta. When converted, he became famous for his liberality in almsgiving.]

[Footnote 2: "Samadhi," says Eitel, "signifies the highest pitch of abstract, ecstatic meditation; a state of absolute indifference to all influences from within or without; a state of torpor of both the material and spiritual forces of vitality; a sort of terrestrial Nirvana, consistently culminating in total destruction of life."]

CHAPTER XXVII

King Asoka's Spirit-built Palace and Halls

Having crossed the river, and descended south for a yojana, the travellers came to the town of Pataliputtra [1], in the kingdom of Magadha, the city where king Asoka ruled. The royal palace and halls in the midst of the city, which exist now as of old, were all made by spirits which he employed, and which piled up the stones, reared the walls and gates, and executed the elegant carving and inlaid sculpture-work—in a way which no human hands of this world could accomplish.

King Asoka had a younger brother who had attained to be an Arhat, and resided on Gridhra-kuta hill, finding his delight in solitude and quiet. The king, who sincerely reverenced him, wished and begged him to come and live in his family, where he could supply all his wants. The other, however, through his delight in the stillness of the mountain, was unwilling to accept the invitation, on which the king said to him, "Only accept my invitation, and I will make a hill for you inside the city." Accordingly, he provided the materials of a feast, called to him the spirits, and announced to them, "Tomorrow you will all receive my invitation; but as there are no mats for you to sit on, let each one bring his own seat." Next day the spirits came, each one bringing with him a great rock, like a wall, four or five paces square, for a seat. When their sitting was over, the king made them form a hill with the large stones piled on one another, and also at the foot of the hill, with five large square stones, to make an apartment, which might be more than thirty cubits long, twenty cubits wide, and more than ten cubits high.

In this city there had resided a great Brahman, named Radha-sami, a professor of the mahayana, of clear discernment and much wisdom, who understood everything, living by himself in spotless purity. The king of the country honored and reverenced him, and served him as his teacher. If he went to inquire for and greet him, the king did not presume to sit down alongside of him; and if, in his love and reverence, he took hold of his hand, as soon as he let it go, the Brahman made haste to pour water on it and wash it. He might be more than fifty years old, and all the kingdom looked up to him. By means of this one man, the Law of Buddha was widely made-known, and the followers of other doctrines did not find it in their power to persecute the body of monks in any way.

By the side of the tope of Asoka, there has been made a mahayana monastery, very grand and beautiful; there is also a hinayana one; the two together containing six hundred or seven hundred monks. The rules of demeanor and the scholastic arrangements in them are worthy of observation.

Shamans of the highest virtue from all quarters, and students, inquirers wishing to find out truth and the grounds of it, all resort to these monasteries. There also resides in this monastery a Brahman teacher, whose name also is Manjusri, whom the Shamans of greatest virtue in the kingdom, and the mahayana Bhikshus honor and look up to.

The cities and towns of this country are the greatest of all in the Middle Kingdom. The inhabitants are rich and prosperous, and vie with one another in the practice of benevolence and righteousness. Every year on the eighth day of the second month they celebrate a procession of images. They make a four-wheeled car, and on it erect a structure of five stories by means of bamboos tied together. This is supported by a king-post, with poles and lances slanting from it, and is rather more than twenty cubits high, having the shape of a tope. White and silk-like cloth of hair is wrapped all round it, which is then painted in various colors. They make figures of devas, with gold, silver, and lapis lazuli grandly blended and having silken streamers and canopies hung out over them. On the four sides are niches, with a Buddha seated in each, and a Bodhisattva standing in attendance on him. There may be twenty cars, all grand and imposing, but each one different from the others. On the day mentioned, the monks and laity within the borders all come together; they have singers and skilful musicians: they say their devotions with flowers and incense. The Brahmans come and invite the Buddhas to enter the city. These do so in order, and remain two nights in it. All through the night they keep lamps burning, have skilful music, and present offerings. This is the practice in all the other kingdoms as well. The Heads of the Vaisya families in them establish in the cities houses for dispensing charity and medicines. All the poor and destitute in the country, orphans, widowers, and childless men, maimed people and cripples, and all who are diseased, go to those houses, and are provided with every kind of help, and doctors examine their diseases. They get the food and medicines which their cases require, and are made to feel at ease; and when they are better, they go away of themselves.

When king Asoka destroyed the seven topes, intending to make eighty-four thousand, the first which he made was the great tope, more than three li to the south of this city. In front of this there is a footprint of Buddha, where a vihara has been built. The door of it faces the north, and on the south of it there is a stone pillar, fourteen or fifteen cubits in circumference, and more than thirty cubits high, on which there is an inscription, saying, "Asoka gave the Jambudvipa to the general body of all the monks, and then redeemed it from them with money. This he did three times." North from the tope three hundred or four hundred paces, king Asoka built the city of Ne-le. In it there is a stone pillar, which also is more than thirty feet high, with a lion on the top of it. On the pillar there is an inscription recording the things which led to the building of Ne-le, with the number of the year, the day, and the month.

[Footnote 1: The modern Patna. The Sanscrit name means "The city of flowers." It is the Indian Florence.]

CHAPTER XXVIII

Rajagriha, New and Old—Legends Connected with It

The travellers went on from this to the southeast for nine yojanas, and came to a small solitary rocky hill, at the head or end of which was an apartment of stone, facing the south—the place where Buddha sat, when Sakra, Ruler of Devas, brought the deva-musician, Panchasikha, to give pleasure to him by playing on his lute. Sakra then asked Buddha about forty-two subjects, tracing the questions out with his finger one by one on the rock. The prints of his tracing are still there; and here also there is a monastery.

A yojana southwest from this place brought them to the village of Nala, where Sariputtra was born, and to which also he returned, and attained here his pari-nirvana. Over the spot where his body was burned there was built a tope, which is still in existence.

Another yojana to the west brought them to New Rajagriha—the new city which was built by king Ajatasatru. There were two monasteries in it. Three hundred paces outside the west gate, king Ajatasatru, having obtained one portion of the relics of Buddha, built over them a tope, high, large, grand, and beautiful. Leaving the city by the south gate, and proceeding south four li, one enters a valley, and comes to a circular space formed by five hills, which stand all round it, and have the appearance of the suburban wall of a city. Here was the old city of king Bimbisara; from east to west about five or six li, and from north to south seven or eight. It was here that Sariputtra and Maudgalyayana first saw Upasena [1]; that the Nirgrantha made a pit of fire and poisoned the rice, and then invited Buddha to eat with him; that king Ajatasatru made a black elephant intoxicated with liquor, wishing him to injure Buddha; and that at the northeast corner of the city in a large curving space Jivaka built a vihara in the garden of Ambapali, and invited Buddha with his one thousand two hundred and fifty disciples to it, that he might there make his offerings to support them. These places are still there as of old, but inside the city all is emptiness and desolation; no man dwells in it.

[Footnote 1: One of the five first followers of Sakyamuni. He is also called Asvajit; in Pali Assaji; but Asvajit seems to be a military title, "Master or trainer of horses." The two more famous disciples met him, not to lead him, but to be directed by him, to Buddha.]

CHAPTER XXIX

Fa-Hien Passes a Night on Gridhra-kuta Hill

Entering the valley, and keeping along the mountains on the southeast, after ascending fifteen li, the travellers came to mount Gridhra-kuta. Three li before you reach the top, there is a cavern in the rocks, facing the south, in which Buddha sat in meditation. Thirty paces to the northwest there is another, where Ananda was sitting in meditation, when the deva Mara Pisuna, having assumed the form of a large vulture, took his place in front of the cavern, and frightened the disciple. Then Buddha, by his mysterious, supernatural power, made a cleft in the rock, introduced his hand, and stroked Ananda's shoulder, so that his fear immediately passed away. The footprints of the bird and the cleft for Buddha's hand are still there, and hence comes the name of "The Hill of the Vulture Cavern."

In front of the cavern there are the places where the four Buddhas sat. There are caverns also of the Arhats, one where each sat and meditated, amounting to several hundred in all. At the place where in front of his rocky apartment Buddha was walking from east to west in meditation, and Devadatta, from among the beetling cliffs on the north of the mountain, threw a rock across, and hurt Buddha's toes, the rock is still there.

The hall where Buddha preached his Law has been destroyed, and only the foundations of the brick walls remain. On this hill the peak is beautifully green, and rises grandly up; it is the highest of all the five hills. In the New City Fa-hien bought incense-sticks, flowers, oil and lamps, and hired two bhikshus, long resident at the place, to carry them to the peak. When he himself got to it, he made his offerings with the flowers and incense, and lighted the lamps when the darkness began to come on. He felt melancholy, but restrained his tears and said, "Here Buddha delivered the Surangama Sutra. I, Fa-hien, was born when I could not meet with Buddha; and now I only see the footprints which he has left, and the place where he lived, and nothing more." With this, in front of the rock cavern, he chanted the Surangama Sutra, remained there over the night, and then returned towards the New City.

CHAPTER XXX

Srataparna Cave, or Cave of the First Council

Out from the old city, after walking over three hundred paces, on the west of the road, the travellers found the Karanda Bamboo garden, where the old vihara is still in existence, with a company of monks, who keep the ground about it swept and watered.

North of the vihara two or three li there was the Smasanam, which name means in Chinese "the field of graves into which the dead are thrown."

As they kept along the mountain on the south, and went west for three hundred paces, they found a dwelling among the rocks, named the Pippala cave, in which Buddha regularly sat in meditation after taking his mid-day meal.

Going on still to the west for five or six li, on the north of the hill, in the shade, they found the cavern called Srataparna, [1] the place where, after the nirvana of Buddha, five hundred Arhats collected the Sutras. When they brought the Sutras forth, three lofty seats had been prepared and grandly ornamented. Sariputtra occupied the one on the left, and Maudgalyayana that on the right. Of the number of five hundred one was wanting. Mahakasyapa was president on the middle seat. Ananda was then outside the door, and could not get in. At the place there was subsequently raised a tope, which is still existing.

Along the sides of the hill, there are also a very great many cells among the rocks, where the various Arhans sat and meditated. As you leave the old city on the north, and go down east for three li, there is the rock dwelling of Devadatta, and at a distance of fifty paces from it there is a large, square, black rock. Formerly there was a bhikshu, who, as he walked backwards and forwards upon it, thought with himself:—"This body is impermanent, a thing of bitterness and vanity, and which cannot be looked on as pure. I am weary of this body, and troubled by it as an evil." With this he grasped a knife, and was about to kill himself. But he thought again:—"The World-honored one laid down a prohibition against one's killing himself." [2] Further it occurred to him:—"Yes, he did; but I now only wish to kill three poisonous thieves." Immediately with the knife he cut his throat. With the first gash into the flesh he attained the state of a Srotapanna; when he had gone half through, he attained to be an Anagamin; and when he had cut right through, he was an Arhat, and attained to pari-nirvana, and died.

[Footnote 1: A very great place in the annals of Buddhism. The Council in the Srataparna cave did not come together fortuitously, but appears to have been convoked by the older members to settle the rules and doctrines of the order. The cave was prepared for the occasion by king Ajatasatru.]

[Footnote 2: Buddha made a law forbidding the monks to commit suicide. He prohibited any one from discoursing on the miseries of life in such a manner as to cause desperation.]

CHAPTER XXXI

Sakyamuni's Attaining to the Buddhaship

From this place, after travelling to the west for four yojanas, the pilgrims came to the city of Gaya; but inside the city all was emptiness and desolation. Going on again to the south for twenty li, they arrived at the place where the Bodhisattva for six years practised with himself painful austerities. All around was forest.

Three li west from here they came to the place where, when Buddha had gone into the water to bathe, a deva bent down the branch of a tree, by means of which he succeeded in getting out of the pool.

Two li north from this was the place where the Gramika girls presented to Buddha the rice-gruel made with milk; and two li north from this was the place where, seated on a rock under a great tree, and facing the east, he ate the gruel. The tree and the rock are there at the present day. The rock may be six cubits in breadth and length, and rather more than two cubits in height. In Central India the cold and heat are so equally tempered that trees live for several thousand and even for ten thousand years.

Half a yojana from this place to the northeast there was a cavern in the rocks, into which the Bodhisattva entered, and sat cross-legged with his face to the west. As he did so, he said to himself, "If I am to attain to perfect wisdom and become Buddha, let there be a supernatural attestation of it." On the wall of the rock there appeared immediately the shadow of a Buddha, rather more than three feet in length, which is still bright at the present day. At this moment heaven and earth were greatly moved, and devas in the air spoke plainly, "This is not the place where any Buddha of the past, or he that is to come, has attained, or will attain, to perfect Wisdom. Less than half a yojana from this to the southwest will bring you to the patra tree, where all past Buddhas have attained, and all to come must attain, to perfect Wisdom." When they had spoken these words, they immediately led the way forward to the place, singing as they did so. As they thus went away, the Bodhisattva arose and walked after them. At a distance of thirty paces from the tree, a deva gave him the grass of lucky omen, which he received and went on. After he had proceeded fifteen paces, five hundred green birds came flying towards him, went round him thrice, and disappeared. The Bodhisattva went forward to the patra tree, placed the kusa grass at the foot of it, and sat down with his face to the east. Then king Mara sent three beautiful young ladies, who came from the north, to tempt him, while he himself came from the south to do the same. The Bodhisattva put his toes down on the ground, and the demon soldiers retired and dispersed, and the three young ladies were changed into old grandmothers.

At the place mentioned above of the six years' painful austerities, and at all these other places, men subsequently reared topes and set up images, which all exist at the present day.

Where Buddha, after attaining to perfect Wisdom, for seven days contemplated the tree, and experienced the joy of vimukti; where, under the patra tree, he walked to and fro from west to east for seven days; where the devas made a hall appear, composed of the seven precious substances, and presented offerings to him for seven days; where the blind dragon Muchilinda [1] encircled him for seven days; where he sat under the nyagrodha tree, on a square rock, with his face to the east, and Brahma-deva came and made his request to him; where the four deva kings brought to him their alms-bowls; where the five hundred merchants presented to him the roasted flour and honey; and where he converted the brothers Kasyapa and their thousand disciples;—at all these places topes were reared.

At the place where Buddha attained to perfect Wisdom, there are three monasteries, in all of which there are monks residing. The families of their people around supply the societies of these monks with an abundant sufficiency of what they require, so that there is no lack or stint. The disciplinary rules are strictly observed by them. The laws regulating their demeanor in sitting, rising, and entering when the others are assembled, are those which have been practised by all the saints since Buddha was in the world down to the present day. The places of the four great topes have been fixed, and handed down without break, since Buddha attained to nirvana. Those four great topes are those at the places where Buddha was born; where he attained to Wisdom; where he began to move the wheel of his Law; and where he attained to pari-nirvana.

[Footnote 1: Called also Maha, or the Great Muchilinda. Eitel says: "A naga king, the tutelary deity of a lake near which Sakyamuni once sat for seven days absorbed in meditation, whilst the king guarded him." The account in "The Life of the Buddha" is:—"Buddha went to where lived the naga king Muchilinda, and he, wishing to preserve him from the sun and rain, wrapped his body seven times round him, and spread out his hood over his head; and there he remained seven days in thought."]

CHAPTER XXXII

Legend of King Asoka in a Former Birth

When king Asoka, in a former birth, was a little boy and playing on the road, he met Kasyapa Buddha walking. The stranger begged food, and the boy pleasantly took a handful of earth and gave it to him. The Buddha took the earth, and returned it to the ground on which he was walking; but because of this the boy received the recompense of becoming a king of the iron wheel, to rule over Jambudvipa. Once when he was making a judicial tour of inspection through Jambudvipa, he saw, between the iron circuit of the two hills, a naraka for the punishment of wicked men. Having thereupon asked his ministers what sort of a thing it was, they replied, "It belongs to Yama, [1] king of demons, for punishing wicked people." The king thought within himself:—"Even the king of demons is able to make a naraka in which to deal with wicked men; why should not I, who am the lord of men, make a naraka in which to deal with wicked men?" He forthwith asked his ministers who could make for him a naraka and preside over the punishment of wicked people in it. They replied that it was only a man of extreme wickedness who could make it; and the king thereupon sent officers to seek everywhere for such a bad man; and they saw by the side of a pond a man tall and strong, with a black countenance, yellow hair, and green eyes, hooking up the fish with his feet, while he called to him birds and beasts, and, when they came, then shot and killed them, so that not one escaped. Having got this man, they took him to the king, who secretly charged him, "You must make a square enclosure with high walls. Plant in it all kinds of flowers and fruits; make good ponds in it for bathing; make it grand and imposing in every way, so that men shall look to it with thirsting desire; make its gates strong and sure; and when any one enters, instantly seize him and punish him as a sinner, not allowing him to get out. Even if I should enter, punish me as a sinner in the same way, and do not let me go. I now appoint you master of that naraka."

Soon after this a bhikshu, pursuing his regular course of begging his food, entered the gate of the place. When the lictors of the naraka saw him, they were about to subject him to their tortures; but he, frightened, begged them to allow him a moment in which to eat his mid-day meal. Immediately after, there came in another man, whom they thrust into a mortar and pounded till a red froth overflowed. As the bhikshu looked on, there came to him the thought of the impermanence, the painful suffering and inanity of this body, and how it is but as a bubble and as foam; and instantly he attained to Arhatship. Immediately after, the lictors seized him, and threw him into a caldron of boiling water. There was a look of joyful satisfaction, however, in the bhikshu's countenance. The fire was extinguished, and the water became cold. In the middle of the caldron there rose up a lotus flower, with the bhikshu seated on it. The lictors at once went and reported to the king that there was a marvellous occurrence in the naraka, and wished him to go and see it; but the king said, "I formerly made such an agreement that now I dare not go to the place." The lictors said, "This is not a small matter. Your Majesty ought to go quickly. Let your former agreement be altered." The king thereupon followed them, and entered the naraka, when the bhikshu preached the Law to him, and he believed, and was made free. Forthwith he demolished the naraka, and repented of all the evil which he had formerly done. From this time he believed in and honored the Three Precious Ones, and constantly went to a patra tree, repenting under it, with self-reproach, of his errors, and accepting the eight rules of abstinence.

The queen asked where the king was constantly going to, and the ministers replied that he was constantly to be seen under such and such a patra tree. She watched for a time when the king was not there, and then sent men to cut the tree down. When the king came, and saw what had been done, he swooned away with sorrow, and fell to the ground. His ministers sprinkled water on his face, and after a considerable time he revived. He then built all round the stump with bricks, and poured a hundred pitchers of cows' milk on the roots; and as he lay with his four limbs spread out on the ground, he took this oath, "If the tree do not live, I will never rise from this." When he had uttered this oath, the tree immediately began to grow from the roots, and it has continued to grow till now, when it is nearly one hundred cubits in height.

[Footnote 1: Yama was originally the Aryan god of the dead, living in a heaven above the world, the regent of the south; but Brahmanism transferred his abode to hell. Both views have been retained by Buddhism. The Yama of the text is the "regent of the narakas, residing south of Jambudvipa, outside the Chakravalas (the double circuit of mountains above), in a palace built of brass and iron. He has a sister who controls all the female culprits, as he exclusively deals with the male sex. Three times, however, in every twenty-four hours, a demon pours boiling copper into Yama's mouth, and squeezes it down his throat, causing him unspeakable pain." Such, however, is the wonderful "transrotation of births," that when Yama's sins have been expiated, he is to be reborn as Buddha, under the name of "The Universal King."]

CHAPTER XXXIII

Kasyapa Buddha's Skeleton on Mount Gurupada

The travellers, going on from this three li to the south, came to a mountain named Gurupada, inside which Mahakasyapa even now is. He made a cleft, and went down into it, though the place where he entered would not now admit a man. Having gone down very far, there was a hole on one side, and there the complete body of Kasyapa still abides. Outside the hole at which he entered is the earth with which he had washed his hands. If the people living thereabouts have a sore on their heads, they plaster on it some of the earth from this, and feel immediately easier. On this mountain, now as of old, there are Arhats abiding. Devotees of our Law from the various countries in that quarter go year by year to the mountain, and present offerings to Kasyapa; and to those whose hearts are strong in faith there come Arhats at night, and talk with them, discussing and explaining their doubts, and disappearing suddenly afterwards.

On this hill hazels grow luxuriantly; and there are many lions, tigers, and wolves, so that people should not travel incautiously.

CHAPTER XXXIV

On the Way Returning to Patna

Fa-Hien returned from here towards Pataliputtra, keeping along the course of the Ganges and descending in the direction of the west. After going ten yojanas he found a vihara, named "The Wilderness"—a place where Buddha had dwelt, and where there are monks now.

Pursuing the same course, and going still to the west, he arrived, after twelve yojanas, at the city of Varanasi in the kingdom of Kasi. Rather more than ten li to the northeast of the city, he found the vihara in the park of "The rishi's Deer-wild." [1] In this park there formerly resided a Pratyeka Buddha, with whom the deer were regularly in the habit of stopping for the night. When the World-honored one was about to attain to perfect Wisdom, the devas sang in the sky, "The son of king Suddhodana, having quitted his family and studied the Path of Wisdom, will now in seven days become Buddha." The Pratyeka Buddha heard their words, and immediately attained to nirvana; and hence this place was named "The Park of the rishi's Deer-wild." After the World-honored one had attained to perfect Wisdom, men built the vihara in it.

Buddha wished to convert Kaundinya and his four companions; but they, being aware of his intention, said to one another, "This Sramana Gotama [2] for six years continued in the practice of painful austerities, eating daily only a single hemp-seed, and one grain of rice, without attaining to the Path of Wisdom; how much less will he do so now that he has entered again among men, and is giving the reins to the indulgence of his body, his speech, and his thoughts! What has he to do with the Path of Wisdom? To-day, when he comes to us, let us be on our guard not to speak with him." At the places where the five men all rose up, and respectfully saluted Buddha, when he came to them; where, sixty paces north from this, he sat with his face to the east, and first turned the wheel of the Law, converting Kaundinya and the four others; where, twenty paces further to the north, he delivered his prophecy concerning Maitreya; and where, at a distance of fifty paces to the south, the dragon Elapattra asked him, "When shall I get free from this naga body?"—at all these places topes were reared, and are still existing. In the park there are two monasteries, in both of which there are monks residing.

When you go northwest from the vihara of the Deer-wild park for thirteen yojanas, there is a kingdom named Kausambi. Its vihara is named Ghochiravana—a place where Buddha formerly resided. Now, as of old, there is a company of monks there, most of whom are students of the hinayana.

East from this, when you have travelled eight yojanas, is the place where Buddha converted the evil demon. There, and where he walked in meditation and sat at the place which was his regular abode, there have been topes erected. There is also a monastery, which may contain more than a hundred monks.

[Footnote 1: "The rishi," says Eitel, "is a man whose bodily frame has undergone a certain transformation by dint of meditation and asceticism, so that he is, for an indefinite period, exempt from decrepitude, age, and death. As this period is believed to extend far beyond the usual duration of human life, such persons are called, and popularly believed to be, immortals." Rishis are divided into various classes; and rishi-ism is spoken of as a seventh path of transrotation, and rishis are referred to as the seventh class of sentient beings.]

[Footnote 2: This is the only instance in Fa-hien's text where the Bodhisattva or Buddha is called by the surname "Gotama." For the most part our traveller uses Buddha as a proper name, though it properly means "The Enlightened." He uses also the combinations "Sakya Buddha," which means "The Buddha of the Sakya tribe," and "Sakyamuni," which means "The Sakya sage." This last is the most common designation of the Buddha in China. Among other Buddhistic peoples "Gotama" and "Gotama Buddha" are the more frequent designations.]

CHAPTER XXXV

Dakshina, and the Pigeon Monastery

South from this two hundred yojanas, there is a country named Dakshina, where there is a monastery dedicated to the by-gone Kasyapa Buddha, and which has been hewn out from a large hill of rock. It consists in all of five stories;—the lowest, having the form of an elephant, with five hundred apartments in the rock; the second, having the form of a lion, with four hundred apartments; the third, having the form of a horse, with three hundred apartments; the fourth, having the form of an ox, with two hundred apartments; and the fifth, having the form of a pigeon, with one hundred apartments. At the very top there is a spring, the water of which, always in front of the apartments in the rock, goes round among the rooms, now circling, now curving, till in this way it arrives at the lowest story, having followed the shape of the structure, and flows out there at the door. Everywhere in the apartments of the monks, the rock has been pierced so as to form windows for the admission of light, so that they are all bright, without any being left in darkness. At the four corners of the tiers of apartments, the rock has been hewn so as to form steps for ascending to the top of each. The men of the present day, being of small size, and going up step by step, manage to get to the top; but in a former age they did so at one step. Because of this, the monastery is called Paravata, that being the Indian name for a pigeon. There are always Arhats residing in it.

The country about is a tract of uncultivated hillocks, without inhabitants. At a very long distance from the hill there are villages, where the people all have bad and erroneous views, and do not know the Sramanas of the Law of Buddha, Brahmanas, or devotees of any of the other and different schools. The people of that country are constantly seeing men on the wing, who come and enter this monastery. On one occasion, when devotees of various countries came to perform their worship at it, the people of those villages said to them, "Why do you not fly? The devotees whom we have seen hereabouts all fly"; and the strangers answered, on the spur of the moment, "Our wings are not yet fully formed."

The kingdom of Dakshina is out of the way, and perilous to traverse. There are difficulties in connection with the roads; but those who know how to manage such difficulties and wish to proceed should bring with them money and various articles, and give them to the king. He will then send men to escort them. These will, at different stages, pass them over to others, who will show them the shortest routes. Fa-hien, however, was after all unable to go there; but having received the above accounts from men of the country, he has narrated them.

CHAPTER XXXVI

Fa-Hien's Indian Studies

From Varanasi the travellers went back east to Pataliputtra. Fa-hien's original object had been to search for copies of the Vinaya. In the various kingdoms of North India, however, he had found one master transmitting orally the rules to another, but no written copies which he could transcribe. He had therefore travelled far and come on to Central India. Here, in the mahayana monastery, he found a copy of the Vinaya, containing the Mahasanghika [1] rules—those which were observed in the first Great Council, while Buddha was still in the world. The original copy was handed down in the Jetavana vihara. As to the other eighteen schools, each one has the views and decisions of its own masters. Those agree with this in the general meaning, but they have small and trivial differences, as when one opens and another shuts. This copy of the rules, however, is the most complete, with the fullest explanations. [2]

He further got a transcript of the rules in six or seven thousand gathas, [3] being the sarvastivadah [4] rules—those which are observed by the communities of monks in the land of Ts'in; which also have all been handed down orally from master to master without being committed to writing. In the community here, moreover, he got the Samyuktabhi-dharma-hridaya-sastra, containing about six or seven thousand gathas; he also got a Sutra of two thousand five hundred gathas; one chapter of the Pari-nirvana-vaipulya Sutra, of about five thousand gathas; and the Mahasanghika Abhidharma.

In consequence of this success in his quest Fa-hien stayed here for three years, learning Sanscrit books and the Sanscrit speech, and writing out, the Vinaya rules. When Tao-ching arrived in the Central Kingdom, and saw the rules observed by the Sramanas, and the dignified demeanor in their societies which he remarked under all occurring circumstances, he sadly called to mind in what a mutilated and imperfect condition the rules were among the monkish communities in the land of Ts'in, and made the following aspiration: "From this time forth till I come to the state of Buddha, let me not be born in a frontier-land." He remained accordingly in India, and did not return to the land of Han. Fa-hien, however, whose original purpose had been to secure the introduction of the complete Vinaya rules into the land of Han, returned there alone.

[Footnote 1: Mahasanghika simply means "the Great Assembly," that is, of monks.]

[Footnote 2: It was afterwards translated by Fa-hien into Chinese.]

[Footnote 3: A gatha is a stanza, generally consisting of a few, commonly of two, lines somewhat metrically arranged.]

[Footnote 4: "A branch," says Eitel, "of the great vaibhashika school, asserting the reality of all visible phenomena, and claiming the authority of Rahula."]

CHAPTER XXXVII

Fa-hien's Stay in Champa and Tamalipti

Following the course of the Ganges, and descending eastward for eighteen yojanas, he found on the southern bank the great kingdom of Champa, with topes reared at the places where Buddha walked in meditation by his vihara, and where he and the three Buddhas, his predecessors, sat. There were monks residing at them all. Continuing his journey east for nearly fifty yojanas, he came to the country of Tamalipti, the capital of which is a seaport. In the country there are twenty-two monasteries, at all of which there are monks residing. The Law of Buddha is also flourishing in it. Here Fa-hien stayed two years, writing out his Sutras, and drawing pictures of images.

After this he embarked in a large merchant-vessel, and went floating over the sea to the southwest. It was the beginning of winter, and the wind was favorable; and, after fourteen days, sailing day and night, they came to the country of Singhala. The people said that it was distant from Tamalipti about seven hundred yojanas.

The kingdom is on a large island, extending from east to west fifty yojanas, and from north to south thirty. Left and right from it there are as many as one hundred small islands, distant from one another ten, twenty, or even two hundred li; but all subject to the large island. Most of them produce pearls and precious stones of various kinds; there is one which produces the pure and brilliant pearl—an island which would form a square of about ten li. The king employs men to watch and protect it, and requires three out of every ten pearls which the collectors find.

CHAPTER XXXVIII

At Ceylon—Feats of Buddha—His Statue in Jade

The country originally had no human inhabitants, but was occupied only by spirits and nagas, with which merchants of various countries carried on a trade. When the trafficking was taking place, the spirits did not show themselves. They simply set forth their precious commodities, with labels of the price attached to them; while the merchants made their purchases according to the price; and took the things away.

Through the coming and going of the merchants in this way, when they went away, the people of their various countries heard how pleasant the land was, and flocked to it in numbers till it became a great nation. The climate is temperate and attractive, without any difference of summer and winter. The vegetation is always luxuriant. Cultivation proceeds whenever men think fit: there are no fixed seasons for it.

When Buddha came to this country, wishing to transform the wicked nagas by his supernatural power, he planted one foot at the north of the royal city, and the other on the top of a mountain, [1] the two being fifteen yojanas apart. Over the footprint at the north of the city the king built a large tope, four hundred cubits high, grandly adorned with gold and silver, and finished with a combination of all the precious substances. By the side of the tope he further built a monastery, called the Abhayagiri, where there are now five thousand monks. There is in it a hall of Buddha, adorned with carved and inlaid work of gold and silver, and rich in the seven precious substances, in which there is an image of Buddha in green jade, more than twenty cubits in height, glittering all over with those substances, and having an appearance of solemn dignity which words cannot express. In the palm of the right hand there is a priceless pearl. Several years had now elapsed since Fa-hien left the land of Han; the men with whom he had been in intercourse had all been of regions strange to him; his eyes had not rested on an old and familiar hill or river, plant or tree: his fellow-travellers, moreover, had been separated from him, some by death, and others flowing off in different directions; no face or shadow was now with him but his own, and a constant sadness was in his heart. Suddenly one day, when by the side of this image of jade, he saw a merchant presenting as his offering a fan of white silk; [2] and the tears of sorrow involuntarily filled his eyes and fell down.

A former king of the country had sent to Central India and got a slip of the patra tree, which he planted by the side of the hall of Buddha, where a tree grew up to the height of about two hundred cubits. As it bent on one side towards the southeast, the king, fearing it would fall, propped it with a post eight or nine spans around. The tree began to grow at the very heart of the prop, where it met the trunk; a shoot pierced through the post, and went down to the ground, where it entered and formed roots, that rose to the surface and were about four spans round. Although the post was split in the middle, the outer portions kept hold of the shoot, and people did not remove them. Beneath the tree there has been built a vihara, in which there is an image of Buddha seated, which the monks and commonalty reverence and look up to without ever becoming wearied. In the city there has been reared also the vihara of

Buddha's tooth, in which, as well as on the other, the seven precious substances have been employed.

The king practises the Brahmanical purifications, and the sincerity of the faith and reverence of the population inside the city are also great. Since the establishment of government in the kingdom there has been no famine or scarcity, no revolution or disorder. In the treasuries of the monkish communities there are many precious stones, and the priceless manis. One of the kings once entered one of those treasuries, and when he looked all round and saw the priceless pearls, his covetous greed was excited, and he wished to take them to himself by force. In three days, however, he came to himself, and immediately went and bowed his head to the ground in the midst of the monks, to show his repentance of the evil thought. As a sequel to this, he informed the monks of what had been in his mind, and desired them to make a regulation that from that day forth the king should not be allowed to enter the treasury and see what it contained, and that no bhikshu should enter it till after he had been in orders for a period of full forty years.

In the city there are many Vaisya elders and Sabaean merchants, whose houses are stately and beautiful. The lanes and passages are kept in good order. At the heads of the four principal streets there have been built preaching halls, where, on the eighth, fourteenth, and fifteenth days of the month, they spread carpets, and set forth a pulpit, while the monks and commonalty from all quarters come together to hear the Law. The people say that in the kingdom there may be altogether sixty thousand monks, who get their food from their common stores. The king, besides, prepares elsewhere in the city a common supply of food for five or six thousand more. When any want, they take their great bowls, and go to the place of distribution, and take as much as the vessels will hold, all returning with them full.

The tooth of Buddha is always brought forth in the middle of the third month. Ten days beforehand the king grandly caparisons a large elephant, on which he mounts a man who can speak distinctly, and is dressed in royal robes, to beat a large drum, and make the following proclamation: "The Bodhisattva, during three Asankhyeya-kalpas, [3] manifested his activity, and did not spare his own life. He gave up kingdom, city, wife, and son; he plucked out his eyes and gave them to another; he cut off a piece of his flesh to ransom the life of a dove; he cut off his head and gave it as an alms; he gave his body to feed a starving tigress; he grudged not his marrow and brains. In many such ways as these did he undergo pain for the sake of all living. And so it was, that, having become Buddha, he continued in the world for forty-five years, preaching his Law, teaching and transforming, so that those who had no rest found rest, and the unconverted were converted. When his connection with the living was completed, he attained to pari-nirvana and died. Since that event, for one thousand four hundred and ninety-seven years, the light of the world has gone out, and all living things have had long-continued sadness. Behold! ten days after this, Buddha's tooth will be brought forth, and taken to the Abhayagiri -vihara. Let all and each, whether monks or laics, who wish to amass merit for themselves, make the roads smooth and in good condition, grandly adorn the lanes and by-ways, and provide abundant store of flowers and incense to be used as offerings to it."

When this proclamation is over, the king exhibits, so as to line both sides of the road, the five hundred different bodily forms in which the Bodhisattva has in the course of his history appeared:—here as Sudana, there as Sama; now as the king of elephants, and then as a stag or a horse. All these figures are brightly colored and grandly executed, looking as if they were alive. After this the tooth of Buddha is brought forth, and is carried along in the middle of the road. Everywhere on the way offerings are presented to it, and thus it arrives at the hall of Buddha in the Abhayagiri-vihara. There monks and laics are collected in crowds. They burn incense, light lamps, and perform all the prescribed services, day and night without ceasing, till ninety days have been completed, when the tooth is returned to the vihara within the city. On fast-days the door of that vihara is opened, and the forms of ceremonial reverence are observed according to the rules.

Forty li to the east of the Abhayagiri-vihara there is a hill, with a vihara on it, called the Chaitya, where there may be two thousand monks. Among them there is a Sramana of great virtue, named Dharma-gupta, honored and looked up to by all the kingdom. He has lived for more than forty years in an apartment of stone, constantly showing such gentleness of heart, that he has brought snakes and rats to stop together in the same room, without doing one another any harm.

[Footnote 1: This would be what is known as "Adam's peak," having, according to Hardy, the three names of Selesumano, Samastakuta, and Samanila. There is an indentation on the top of it, a superficial hollow, 5 feet 3 3/4 inches long, and 2 1/2 feet wide. The Hindus regard it as the footprint of Siva; the Mohammedans, as that of Adam; and the Buddhists, as in the text—as having been, made by Buddha.]

[Footnote 2: We naturally suppose that the merchant-offerer was a Chinese, as indeed the Chinese texts say, and the fan such as Fa-hien had seen and used in his native land.]

[Footnote 3: A Kalpa, we have seen, denotes a great period of time; a period during which a physical universe is formed and destroyed. Asankhyeya denotes the highest sum for which a conventional term exists—according to Chinese calculations equal to one followed by seventeen ciphers; according to Thibetan and Singhalese, equal to one followed by ninety-seven ciphers. Every Maha-kalpa consists of four Asankhye-yakalpas.]

CHAPTER XXXIX

Cremation of an Arhat—Sermon of a Devotee

South of the city seven li there is a vihara, called the Maha-vihara, where three thousand monks reside. There had been among them a Sramana, of such lofty virtue, and so holy and pure in his observance of the disciplinary rules, that the people all surmised that he was an Arhat. When he drew near his end, the king came to examine into the point; and having assembled the monks according to rule, asked whether the bhikshu had attained to the full degree of Wisdom. They answered in the affirmative, saying that he was an Arhat. The king accordingly, when he died, buried him after the fashion of an Arhat, as the regular rules prescribed. Four or five li east from the vihara there was reared a great pile of firewood, which might be more than thirty cubits square, and the same in height. Near the top were laid sandal, aloe, and other kinds of fragrant wood.

On the four sides of the pile they made steps by which to ascend it. With clean white hair-cloth, almost like silk, they wrapped the body round and round. They made a large carriage-frame, in form like our funeral car, but without the dragons and fishes.

At the time of the cremation, the king and the people, in multitudes from all quarters, collected together, and presented offerings of flowers and incense. While they were following the car to the burial-ground, the king himself presented flowers and incense. When this was finished, the car was lifted on the pile, all over which oil of sweet basil was poured, and then a light was applied. While the fire was blazing, every one, with a reverent heart, pulled off his upper garment, and threw it, with his feather-fan and umbrella, from a distance into the midst of the flames, to assist the burning. When the cremation was over, they collected and preserved the bones, and proceeded to erect a tope. Fa-hien had not arrived in time to see the distinguished Shaman alive, and only saw his burial.

At that time the king, who was a sincere believer in the Law of Buddha and wished to build a new vihara for the monks, first convoked a great assembly. After giving the monks a meal of rice, and presenting his offerings on the occasion, he selected a pair of first-rate oxen, the horns of which were grandly decorated with gold, silver, and the precious substances. A golden plough had been provided, and the king himself turned up a furrow on the four sides of the ground within which the building was to be. He then endowed the community of the monks with the population, fields, and houses, writing the grant on plates of metal, to the effect that from that time onwards, from generation to generation, no one should venture to annul or alter it.

In this country Fa-hien heard an Indian devotee, who was reciting a Sutra from the pulpit, say: "Buddha's alms-bowl was at first in Vaisali, and now it is in Gandhara. After so many hundred years (he gave, when Fa-hien heard him, the exact number of years, but he has forgotten it), it will go to Western Tukhara; after so many hundred years, to Khoten; after so many hundred years, to Kharachar; after so many hundred years, to the land of Han; after so many hundred years, it will come to Sinhala; and after so many hundred years, it will return to Central India. After that, it will ascend to the Tushita heaven; and when the Bodhisattva Maitreya sees it, he will say with a sigh, 'The alms-bowl of Sakyamuni Buddha is come'; and with all the devas he will present to it flowers and incense for seven days. When these have expired, it will return to Jambudvipa, where it will be received by the king of the sea nagas, and taken into his naga palace. When Maitreya shall be about to attain to perfect Wisdom and become Buddha, it will again separate into four bowls, which will return to the top of mount Anna, whence they came. After Maitreya has become Buddha, the four deva kings will again think of the Buddha with their bowls as they did in the case of the previous Buddha. The thousand Buddhas of this Bhadra-kalpa, indeed, will all use the same alms-bowl; and when the bowl has disappeared, the Law of Buddha will go on gradually to be extinguished. After that extinction has taken place, the life of man will be shortened, till it is only a period of five years. During this period of a five years' life, rice, butter, and oil will all vanish away, and men will become exceedingly wicked. The grass and trees which they lay hold of will change into swords and clubs, with which they will hurt, cut, and kill one another. Those among them on whom there is blessing will withdraw from society among the hills; and when the wicked have exterminated one another, they will again come forth, and say among themselves, 'The men of former times enjoyed a very great longevity; but through becoming exceedingly wicked, and doing all lawless things, the length of our life has been shortened and reduced even to five years. Let us now unite together in the practice of what is good, cherishing a gentle and sympathizing heart, and carefully cultivating good faith and righteousness. When each one in this way practises that faith and righteousness, life will go on to double its length till it reaches eighty thousand years. When Maitreya appears in the world, and begins to turn the wheel of this Law, he will in the first place save those among the disciples of the Law left by the Sakya who have quitted their families, and those who have accepted the three Refuges, undertaken the five Prohibitions and the eight Abstinences, and given offerings to the Three Precious Ones; secondly and thirdly, he will save those between whom and conversion there is a connection transmitted from the past.'" [1]

Such was the discourse, and Fa-hien wished to write it down as a portion of doctrine; but the man said, "This is taken from no Sutra, it is only the utterance of my own mind."

[Footnote 1: That is, those whose Karma in the past should be rewarded by such conversion in the present.]

CHAPTER XL

After Two Years Fa-hien Takes Ship for China

Fa-hien abode in this country two years; and, in addition to his acquisitions in Patna, succeeded in getting a copy of the Vinaya-pitaka of the Mahisasakah school; the Dirghagama and Samyuktagama Sutras; and also the Samyukta-sanchaya-pitaka;—all being works unknown in the land of Han. Having obtained these Sanscrit works, he took passage in a large merchantman, on board of which there were more than two hundred men, and to which was attached by a rope a smaller vessel, as a provision against damage or injury to the large one from the perils of the navigation. With a favorable wind, they proceeded eastward for three days, and then they encountered a great wind. The vessel sprang a leak and the water came in. The merchants wished to go to the smaller vessel; but the men on board it, fearing that too many would come, cut the connecting rope. The merchants were greatly alarmed, feeling their risk of instant death. Afraid that the vessel would fill, they took their bulky goods and threw them into the water. Fa-hien also took his pitcher and washing-basin, with some other articles, and cast them into the sea; but fearing that the merchants would cast overboard his books and images, he could only think with all his heart of Kwan-she-yin, and commit his life to the protection of the church of the land of Han, saying in effect, "I have travelled far in search of our Law. Let me, by your dread and supernatural power, return from my wanderings, and reach my resting-place!"

In this way the tempest continued day and night, till on the thirteenth day the ship was carried to the side of an island, where, on the ebbing of the tide, the place of the leak was discovered, and it was stopped, on which the voyage was resumed. On the sea hereabouts there are many pirates, to meet with whom is speedy death. The great ocean spreads out, a boundless expanse. There is no knowing east or west; only by observing the sun, moon, and stars was it possible to go forward. If the weather were dark and rainy, the ship went as she was carried by the wind, without any definite course. In the darkness of the night, only the great waves were to be seen, breaking on one another, and emitting a brightness like that of fire, with huge turtles and other monsters of the deep all about. The merchants were full of terror, not knowing where they were going. The sea was deep and bottomless, and there was no place where they could drop anchor and stop. But when the sky became clear, they could tell east and west, and the ship again went forward in the right direction. If she had come on any hidden rock, there would have been no way of escape.

After proceeding in this way for rather more than ninety days, they arrived at a country called Java-dvipa, where various forms of error and Brahmanism are flourishing, while Buddhism in it is not worth speaking of. After staying there for five months, Fa-hien again embarked in another large merchantman, which also had on board more than two hundred men. They carried provisions for fifty days, and commenced the voyage on the sixteenth day of the fourth month.

Fa-hien kept his retreat on board the ship. They took a course to the northeast, intending to fetch Kwang-chow. After more than a month, when the night-drum had sounded the second watch, they encountered a black wind and tempestuous rain, which threw the merchants and passengers into consternation. Fa-hien again, with all his heart, directed his thoughts to Kwan-she-yin and the monkish communities of the land of Han; and, through their dread and mysterious protection, was preserved to daybreak. After daybreak, the Brahmans deliberated together and said, "It is having this Sramana on board which has occasioned our misfortune and brought us this great and bitter suffering. Let us land the bhikshu and place him on some island-shore. We must not for the sake of one man allow ourselves to be exposed to such imminent peril." A patron of Fa-hien, however, said to them, "If you land the bhikshu, you must at the same time land me; and if you do not, then you must kill me. If you land this Sramana, when I get to the land of Han, I will go to the king, and inform against you. The king also reveres and believes the Law of Buddha, and honors the bhikshus." The merchants hereupon were perplexed, and did not dare immediately to land Fa-hien.

At this time the sky continued very dark and gloomy, and the sailing-masters looked at one another and made mistakes. More than seventy days passed from their leaving Java, and the provisions and water were nearly exhausted. They used the salt-water of the sea for cooking, and carefully divided the fresh water, each man getting two pints. Soon the whole was nearly gone, and the merchants took counsel and said, "At the ordinary rate of sailing we ought to have reached Kwang-chow, and now the time is passed by many days;—must we not have held a wrong course?" Immediately they directed the ship to the northwest, looking out for land; and after sailing day and night for twelve days, they reached the shore on the south of mount Lao, on the borders of the prefecture of Ch'ang-kwang, and immediately got good water and vegetables. They had passed through many perils and hardships, and had been in a state of anxious apprehension for many days together; and now suddenly arriving at this shore, and seeing those well-known vegetables, the lei and kwoh, [1] they knew indeed that it was the land of Han. Not seeing, however, any inhabitants nor any traces of them, they did not know whereabouts they were. Some said that they had not yet got to Kwang-chow, and others that they had passed it. Unable to come to a definite conclusion, some of them got into a small boat and entered a creek, to look for someone of whom they might ask what the place was. They found two hunters, whom they brought back with them, and then called on Fa-hien to act as interpreter and question them. Fa-hien first spoke assuringly to them, and then slowly and distinctly asked them, "Who are you?" They replied, "We are disciples of Buddha." He then asked, "What are you looking for among these hills?" They began to lie,[2] and said, "To-morrow is the fifteenth day of the seventh month. We wanted to get some peaches to present to Buddha." He asked further, "What country is this?" They replied, "This is the border of the prefecture of Ch'ang-kwang, a part of Ts'ing-chow under the ruling House of Ts'in." When they heard this, the merchants were glad, immediately asked for a portion of their money and goods, and sent men to Ch'ang-kwang city.

The prefect Le E was a reverent believer in the Law of Buddha. When he heard that a Sramana had arrived in a ship across the sea, bringing with him books and images, he immediately came to the sea-shore with an escort to meet the traveller, and receive the books and images, and took them back with him to the seat of his government. On this the merchants went back in the direction of Yang-chow; but when Fa-hien arrived at Ts'ing-chow, the prefect there begged him to remain with him for a winter and a summer. After the summer retreat was ended, Fa-hien, having been separated for a long time from his fellows, wished to hurry to Ch'ang-gan; but as the business which he had in hand was important, he went south to the Capital; and at an interview with the masters there exhibited the Sutras and the collection of the Vinaya which he had procured.

After Fa-hien set out from Ch'ang-gan, it took him six years to reach Central India; stoppages there extended over six years; and on his return it took him three years to reach Ts'ing-chow. The countries through which he passed were a few under thirty. From the sandy desert westwards on to India, the beauty of the dignified demeanor of the monkhood and of the transforming influence of the Law was beyond the power of language fully to describe; and reflecting how our masters had not heard any complete account of them, he therefore went on without regarding his own poor life, or the dangers to be encountered on the sea upon his return, thus incurring hardships and difficulties in a double form. He was fortunate enough, through the dread power of the three Honored Ones, to receive help and protection in his perils; and therefore he wrote out an account of his experiences, that worthy readers might share with him in what he had heard and said.

[Footnote 1: What these vegetables exactly were it is difficult to say; and there are different readings of the characters for kwoh, brings the two names together in a phrase, but the rendering of it is simply "a soup of simples."]

[Footnote 2: It is likely that these men were really hunters; and, when brought before Fa-hien, because he was a Sramana, they thought they would please him by saying they were disciples of Buddha. But what had disciples of Buddha to do with hunting and taking life? They were caught in their own trap, and said they were looking for peaches.]

THE SORROWS OF HAN

[Translated into English by John Francis Davis]

INTRODUCTION

"The Sorrows of Han" is considered by Chinese scholars to be one of the largest tragedies in the whole range of the Chinese drama, which is very voluminous. Although, properly speaking, there are no theatres in China, the Chinese are passionately fond of dramatic representations. Chinese acting is much admired and praised by travellers who are competent to follow the dialogue. The stage is generally a temporary erection improvised in a market-place, and the stage arrangements are of the most primitive character; no scenery is employed, and the actors introduce themselves in a sort of prologue, in which they state the name and character they represent in the drama. They also indicate the place where they are in the story, or the house which they have entered. Yet the Chinese stage has many points in common with that of Ancient Greece. It is supported and controlled by government, and has something of a religious and national character, being particularly employed for popular amusement in the celebration of religious festivals. Only two actors are allowed to occupy the stage at the same time, and this is another point in common with the early Greek drama. The plots or stories of the Chinese plays are simple and effective, and Voltaire is known to have taken the plot of a Chinese drama, as Moliere took a comedy of Plautus, and applied it in writing a drama for the modern French stage. "The Sorrows of Han" belongs to the famous collection entitled "The Hundred Plays of the Yuen Dynasty." It is divided into acts and is made up of alternate prose and verse. The movement of the drama is good, and the denouement arranged with considerable skill.

E.W.

TRANSLATOR'S PREFACE

The following drama was selected from the "Hundred Plays of Yuen," which has already supplied to Europe two specimens of the Chinese stage—the first, called the "Orphan of Chaou," translated by Pere Premare; and the second, entitled an "Heir in Old Age," by the author of the present version. "The Sorrows of Han" is historical, and relates to one of the most interesting periods of the Chinese annals, when the growing effeminacy of the court, and consequent weakness of the government, emboldened the Tartars in their aggressions, and first gave rise to the temporizing and impolitic system of propitiating those barbarians by tribute, which long after produced the downfall of the empire and the establishment of the Mongol dominion.

The moral of the piece is evidently to expose the evil consequences of luxury, effeminacy, and supineness in the sovereign.

"When love was all an easy monarch's care,
Seldom at council—never in a war."

The hero, or rather the chief personage, of the drama, came to the throne very near the beginning of the Christian era, about B.C. 42. The fate of the Lady Chaoukeun is a favorite incident in history, of which painters, poets, and romancers frequently avail themselves; her "Verdant Lamb" is said to exist at the present day, and to remain green all the year round, while the vegetation of the desert in which it stands is parched by the summer sun.

In selecting this single specimen from among so many, the translator was influenced by the consideration of its remarkable accordance with our own canons of criticism. The Chinese themselves make no regular classification of comedy and tragedy; but we are quite at liberty to give the latter title to a play which so completely answers to the European definition. The unity of action is complete, and the unities of time and place much less violated than they frequently are on our own stage. The grandeur and gravity of the subject, the rank and dignity of the personages, the tragical catastrophe, and the strict award of poetical justice, might satisfy the most rigid admirer of Grecian rules. The translator has thought it necessary to adhere to the original by distinguishing the first act (or Proem) from the four which follow it: but the distinction is purely nominal, and the piece consists, to all intents and purposes, of five acts. It is remarkable that this peculiar division holds true with regard to a large number of the "Hundred Plays of Yuen."

The reader will doubtless be struck by the apparent shortness of the drama which is here presented to him; but the original is eked out, in common with all Chinese plays, by an irregular operatic species of song, which the principal character occasionally chants forth in unison with a louder or a softer accompaniment of music, as may best suit the sentiment or action of the moment. Some passages have been embodied in our version: but the translator did not give all, for the same reasons that prompted Pere Premare to give none—"they are full of allusions to things unfamiliar to us, and figures of speech very difficult for us to observe." They are frequently, moreover, mere repetitions or amplifications of the prose parts; and being intended more for the ear than the eye, are rather adapted to the stage than to the closet.

His judgment may perhaps be swayed by partiality towards the subject of his own labors; but the translator cannot help thinking the plot and incidents of "The Sorrows of Han" superior to those of the "Orphan of Chaou"—though the genius of Voltaire contrived to make the last the ground-work of an excellent French tragedy. Far is he, however, from entertaining the presumptuous expectation that a destiny of equal splendor awaits the present drama; and he will be quite satisfied if the reader has patience to read it to the end, and then pronounces it to be a somewhat curious sample of a very foreign literature.

JOHN FRANCIS DAVIS.

DRAMATIS PERSONAE

YUENTE, Emperor of China of the Dynasty Han.
HANCHENYU, K'han of the Tartars.
MAOUYENSHOW, a worthless Minister of the Emperor.
SHANGSHOO (a title), President of the Imperial Council.
CHANGSHEE (a title), Officer in waiting.
FANSHE (a title), Envoy of the K'han.
CHAOUKEUN, Lady, raised to be Princess of Han.
Tartar Soldiers, Female Attendants, Eunuchs.

The Scene is laid in the Tartar Camp on the Frontiers; and in the Palace of Han.

THE SORROWS OF HAN [1]

PROLOGUE

Enter Hanchenyu, K'han [2] of the Tartars, reciting four verses.

K'HAN. The autumnal gale blows wildly through the grass, amidst our woolen tents.
And the moon of night, shining on the rude huts, hears the lament of the mournful pipe:
The countless hosts, with their bended horns, obey me as their leader.

Our tribes are ten distinguished friends of the family of Han. I am Hanchenyu, the old inhabitant of the sandy waste; the sole ruler of the northern regions. The wild chase is our trade; battle and conquest our chief occupation. The Emperor Wunwong retired before our Eastern tribes; Weikeang trembled at us, and sued for our friendship. The ancient title of our chiefs has in the course of time been changed to that which I now bear. When the two races of Tsin and Han contended in battle, and filled the empire with tumult, our tribes were in full power: numberless was the host of armed warriors with their bended horns. For seven days my ancestor hemmed in with his forces the Emperor Kaoute; until, by the contrivance of the minister, a treaty was concluded, and the Princesses of China were yielded in marriage to our K'hans. Since the time of Hoeyte and the Empress Leuhow, [3] each successive generation has adhered to the established rule, and sought our alliance with its daughters. In the reign of the late Emperor Seuente, my brothers contended with myself for the rule of our nation, and its power was weakened until the tribes elected me as their chief. I am a real descendant of the empire of Han. I command a hundred thousand armed warriors. We have moved to the South, and approached the border, claiming an alliance with the Imperial race. Yesterday I despatched an envoy with tributary presents to demand a princess in marriage; but know not if the Emperor will ratify the engagement with the customary oaths. The fineness of the season has drawn away our chiefs on a hunting excursion amidst the sandy steppes. May they meet with success, for we Tartars have no fields—our bows and arrows are our sole means of subsistence.

Enter Minister of Han, reciting verses.

MINISTER. Let a man have the heart of a kite, and the talons of an eagle.
Let him deceive his superiors, and oppress those below him;
Let him enlist flattery, insinuation, profligacy, and avarice on his side,

And he will find them a lasting assistance through life. I am no other than Maouyenshow, a minister of the sovereign of Han. By a hundred arts of specious flattery and address I have deceived the Emperor, until he places his whole delight in me alone. My words he listens to; and he follows my counsel. Within the precincts of the palace, as without them, who is there but bows before me—who is there but trembles at my approach? But observe the chief art which I have learned: It is this: to persuade the Emperor to keep aloof from his wise counsellors, and seek all his pleasures amidst the women of his palace. Thus it is that I strengthen my power and greatness. But, in the midst of my lucubrations—Here comes the Emperor.

Enter Emperor Yuente, attended by Eunuchs and Women.

EMPEROR [*recites verses]*. During the ten generations that have succeeded our acquisition of Empire, my race has alone possessed the four hundred districts of the world. Long have the frontiers been bound in tranquillity by the ties of mutual oaths. And our pillow has been undisturbed by grief or anxiety. Behold in us the Emperor Yuente, of the race of Han. Our ancestor Kaoute emerged from a private station, and raised his family by extinguishing the dynasty of Tsin, and slaughtering their race. Ten generations have passed away since he left this inheritance to us. The four boundaries of the empire have been tranquil; the eight regions at rest! But not through our personal merits; we have wholly depended on the exertions of our civil and military rulers. On the demise of our late father, the female inmates of the palace were all dispersed, and our harem is now solitary and untenanted; but how shall this be endured!

MINISTER. Consider, sir, that even the thriving husbandman may desire to change his partner; then why not your Majesty, whose title is the Law of Heaven, whose possessions are the whole world! May I advise that commissioners be despatched to search throughout the empire for all of whatever rank that is most beautiful between the ages of fifteen and twenty, for the peopling of the inner palace.

EMPEROR. You say well. We appoint you at once our minister of selection, and will invest you with a written authority. Search diligently through our realms; and when you have selected the most worthy, let us be provided with portraits of each, as a means of fixing our choice. By the merits of your services, you may supply us with an occasion of rewarding you on your return. [*Exeunt.*

[Footnote 1: Han Koong Tsew, literally "Autumn in the Palace of Han"; but in Chinese, Autumn is emblematic of Sorrow, as Spring is of Joy, and may therefore be rendered by what it represents.]

[Footnote 2: In Chinese, Ko-ban.]

[Footnote 3: The mother of Hoeyte, a bold and able woman, who ruled for her son, the second emperor of Han.]

ACT FIRST

MINISTER [*repeats verses*]. The huge ingots of yellow gold I appropriate to myself.
I heed not the seas of blood which flow by perverting the laws.

During life I am determined to have abundance of riches; what care I for the curses of mankind after my death? Having received the Emperor's commission to search far and wide for the most beautiful damsels, I have fixed upon ninety and nine. Their families were glad to invite my selection by rich gifts, and the treasure that I have amassed is not small. On arriving yesterday at a district pertaining to Chingtoo city, I met with a maiden, daughter of one Wongchang. The brightness of her charms was piercing as an arrow. She was perfectly beautiful—and doubtless unparalleled in the whole empire. But, unfortunately, her father is a cultivator of the land, not possessed of much wealth. When I insisted on a hundred ounces of gold to secure her being the chief object of the imperial choice, they first pleaded their poverty—and then, relying on her extraordinary beauty, rejected my offers altogether. I therefore left them. [*Considers awhile.*] But no!——I have a better plan. [*He knits his brows and matures his scheme.*] I will disfigure her portrait in such a manner that when it reaches the Emperor it shall secure her being doomed to neglected seclusion. Thus I shall contrive to make her unhappy for life—Base is the man who delights not in revenge! [*Exit.*

Night.—Enter the Lady Chaoukeun, with two female attendants.

CHAOUKEUN [*recites verses*]. Though raised to be an inhabitant of the imperial dwelling
I have long been here without the good fortune to see my prince.

This beautiful night must I pass in lonely solitude, with no companion but my lute to solace my retirement. I am a native of Chingtoo city; and my father's occupation is husbandry. My mother dreamed on the day I was born that the light of the moon shone on her bosom, but was soon cast low to the earth.[1] I was just eighteen years of age when chosen as an inhabitant of the imperial palace; but the minister Maouyenshow, disappointed in the treasure which he demanded on my account, disfigured my portrait in such a manner as to keep me out of the Emperor's presence; and now I live in neglected solitude. While at home, I learned a little music, and could play a few airs on the lute. Thus sorrowing in the stillness of midnight, let me practise one of my songs to dispel my griefs. [*Begins to play on the lute.*

Enter Emperor, attended by a Eunuch, carrying a light.

EMPEROR. Since the beauties were selected to grace our palace, we have not yet discovered a worthy object on whom to fix our preference. Vexed and disappointed, we pass this day of leisure roaming in search of her who may be destined for our imperial choice. [*Hears the lute.*] Is not that some lady's lute?

ATTENDANT. It is.—I hasten to advise her of your Majesty's approach.

EMPEROR. No, hold! Keeper of the yellow gate, discover to what part of our palace that lady pertains; and bid her approach our presence; but beware lest you alarm her.

ATTENDANT [*approaches in the direction of the sound, and speaks*]. What lady plays there? The Emperor comes! approach to meet him. [*Lady advances.*

EMPEROR. Keeper of the yellow gate, see that the light burns brightly within your gauze [2] lamp, and hold it nearer to us.

LADY [*approaching*]. Had your handmaid but known it was your Majesty, she would have been less tardy; forgive, then, this delay.

EMPEROR. Truly this is a very perfect beauty! From what quarter come such superior charms?

LADY. My name is Chaoukeun: my father cultivates at Chingtoo the fields which he has derived from his family. Born in an humble station, I am ignorant of the manners that befit a palace.

EMPEROR. But with such uncommon attractions, what chance has kept you from our sight?

LADY. When I was chosen by the minister Maouyenshow, he demanded of my father an amount of treasure which our poverty could not supply; he therefore disfigured my portrait, by representing a scar under the eyes, and caused me to be consigned to seclusion and neglect.

EMPEROR. Keeper of the yellow gate, bring us that picture, that we may view it. [*Sees the picture.*] Ah, how has he dimmed the purity of the gem, bright as the waves in autumn. [*To the attendant*] Transmit our pleasure to the officer of the guard, to behead Maouyenshow and report to us his execution.

LADY. My parents, sir, are subject to the tax [3] in our native district. Let me entreat your Majesty to remit their contributions and extend favor towards them!

EMPEROR. That shall readily be done. Approach and hear our imperial pleasure. We create you a Princess of our palace.

LADY. How unworthy is your handmaid of such gracious distinction! [*Goes through the form of returning thanks.*] Early to-morrow I attend your Majesty's commands in this place. The Emperor is gone: let the attendants close the doors:—I will retire to rest. *[Exit.*

[Footnote 1: Boding a short but fatal distinction to her offspring.]

[Footnote 2: Instead of glass, to defend it from the wind.]

[Footnote 3: The principal taxes in China are the land-tax, customs, salt monopoly, and personal service; which last is the source of much oppression to the lowest orders, who have nothing but their labor to contribute.]

ACT SECOND

Enter K'han of the Tartars, at the head of his Tribes.

K'HAN. I lately sent an envoy to the sovereign of Han, with the demand of a princess in marriage; but the Emperor has returned a refusal, under the plea that the princess is yet too young. This answer gives me great trouble. Had he not plenty of ladies in his palace, of whom he might have sent me one? The difference was of little consequence. [1] Let me recall my envoy with all speed, for I must invade the South with out forces. And yet I am unwilling to break a truce of so many years' standing! We must see how matters turn out, and be guided by the event.

Enter Minister of Han.

MINISTER. The severity with which I extorted money, in the selection of beauties for the palace, led me to disfigure the picture of Chaoukeun, and consign her to neglected seclusion. But the Emperor fell in with her, obtained the truth, and condemned me to lose my head. I contrived to make my escape—though I have no home to receive me. I will take this true portrait of Chaoukeun and show it to the Tartar K'han, persuading him to demand her from the Emperor, who will no doubt be obliged to yield her up. A long journey has brought me to this spot, and from the troops of men and horses I conclude I have reached the Tartar camp. [*Addresses himself to somebody*] Leader, inform King Hanchenyu that a great minister of the empire of Han is come to wait on him.

K'HAN [*on being informed*]. Command him to approach. [*Seeing Maouyenshow*] What person are you?

MINISTER. I am a minister of Han. In the western palace of the Emperor is a lady, named Chaoukeun, of rare and surpassing charms. When your envoy, great king, came to demand a princess, this lady would have answered the summons, but the Emperor of Han could not bring himself to part with her, and refused to yield her up. I repeatedly renewed my bitter reproaches, and asked how he could bear, for the sake of a woman's beauty, to implicate the welfare of two nations. For this the Emperor would have beheaded me; and I therefore escaped with the portrait of the lady, which I present, great king, to yourself. Should you send away an envoy with the picture to demand her, she must certainly be delivered up. Here is the portrait. [*Hands it up.*

K'HAN. Whence could so beautiful a female have appeared in the world! If I can only obtain her, my wishes are complete. Immediately shall an envoy be despatched, and my ministers prepare a letter to the Emperor of Han, demanding her in marriage as the condition of peace. Should he refuse, I will presently invade the South: his hills and rivers shall be exposed to ravage. Our warriors will commence by hunting, as they proceed on their way; and thus gradually entering the frontiers, I shall be ready to act as may best suit the occasion. [*Exit.*

The Palace of Han. Enter Lady, attended by females.

PRINCESS. A long period has elapsed since I had to thank his Majesty for his choice. The Emperor's fondness for me is so great, that he has still neglected to hold a court. I hear he is now gone to the hall of audience, and will therefore ornament myself at my toilet and be ready to wait on him at his return. [*Stands opposite a mirror.*

Enter Emperor.

EMPEROR. Since we first met with Chaoukeun in the western palace, we have been as it were deranged and intoxicated; a long interval has elapsed since we held a court; and on entering the hall of audience this day, we waited not until the assembly had dispersed, but returned hither to obtain a sight of her.
[*Perceiving the Princess.*] Let us not alarm her, but observe in secret what she is doing.
[*Comes close behind and looks over her.*] Reflected in that round mirror, she resembles the Lady in the Moon. [2]

Enter President, and an Officer in waiting.

PRESIDENT [*recites verses.*] Ministers should devote themselves to the regulation of the empire; They should be occupied with public cares in the hall of government. But they do nought but attend at the banquets in the palace. When have they employed a single day in the service of their prince?

This day, when the audience was concluded, an envoy arrived from the Tartars to demand Chaoukeun in marriage, as the only condition of peace. It is my duty to report this to his Majesty, who has retired to his western palace. Here I must enter. [*Perceiving the Emperor.*] I report to your Majesty that Hanchenyu, the leader of the northern foreigners, sends an envoy to declare that Maouyenshow has presented to him the portrait of the princess, and that he demands her in marriage as the only condition of peace. If refused, he will invade the South with a great power, and our rivers and hills will be exposed to rapine.

EMPEROR. In vain do we maintain and send forth armies; vain are the crowds of civil and military officers about our palace! Which of them will drive back for us these foreign troops? They are all afraid of the Tartar swords and arrows! But if they cannot exert themselves to expel the barbarians, why call for the princess to propitiate them?

PRESIDENT. The foreigners say that through your Majesty's devoted fondness for the princess, the affairs of your empire are falling into ruin. They declare that if the government does not yield her up, they will put their army in motion, and subdue the country. Your servant reflects, that Chow-wong [3] who lost his empire and life entirely through his blind devotion to Takee, is a fit example to warn your Majesty. Our army is weak, and needs the talents of a fit general. Should we oppose the Tartars, and be defeated, what will remain to us? Let your Majesty give up your fondness for the princess, to save your people.

OFFICER. The envoy waits without for an audience.

EMPEROR. Well; command that he approach us.

Enter Envoy.

ENVOY. Hanchenyu, K'han of the Tartars, sends me, his minister, to state before the great Sovereign of Han, that the Northern tribes and the Southern empire have long been bound in peace by mutual alliances; but that envoys being twice sent to demand a princess, his requisitions have been refused. The late minister, Maouyenshow, took with him the portrait of a beautiful lady, and presented it to the K'ban, who now sends me, his envoy, on purpose to demand the Lady Chaoukeun, and no other, as the only condition of peace between the two nations. Should your Majesty refuse, the K'han has a countless army of brave warriors, and will forthwith invade the South to try the chances of war. I trust your Majesty will not err in your decision.

EMPEROR. The envoy may retire to repose himself in his lodging. [*Exit the Envoy.*] Let our civil and military officers consult, and report to us the best mode of causing the foreign troops to retire, without yielding up the princess to propitiate them. They take advantage of the compliant softness of her temper. Were the Empress Leuhow alive—let her utter a word—which of them would dare to be of a different opinion? It would seem that, for the future, instead of men for ministers, we need only have fair women to keep our empire in peace.

PRINCESS. In return for your Majesty's bounties, it is your handmaid's duty to brave death to serve you. I can cheerfully enter into this foreign alliance, for the sake of producing peace, and shall leave behind me a name still green in history.—But my affection for your Majesty, how am I to lay aside!

EMPEROR. Alas, I [4] know too well that I can do no more than yourself!

PRESIDENT. I entreat your Majesty to sacrifice your love, and think of the security of your Dynasty. Hasten, sir, to send the princess on her way!

EMPEROR. Let her this day advance a stage on her journey, and be presented to the envoy.—To-morrow we will repair as far as the bridge of Pahling, and give her a parting feast.

PRESIDENT. Alas! Sir, this may not be! It will draw on us the contempt of these barbarians.

EMPEROR. We have complied with all our minister's propositions—shall they not, then, accede to ours? Be it as it may, we will witness her departure—and then return home to hate the traitor Maouyenshow!

PRESIDENT. Unwillingly we advise that the princess be sacrificed for the sake of peace; but the envoy is instructed to insist upon her alone—and from ancient times, how often hath a nation suffered for a woman's beauty!

PRINCESS. Though I go into exile for the nation's good, yet ill can I bear to part from your Majesty! *[Exeunt.*

[Footnote 1: The honor of the imperial alliance being the chief object.]

[Footnote 2: Changngo, the goddess of the moon, gives her name to the finely curved eyebrows of the Chinese ladies, which are compared to the lunar crescent when only a day or two old.]

[Footnote 3: Chow-wong was the last of the Shang dynasty, and infamous by his debaucheries and cruelties, in concert with his empress Takee, the Theodora of Chinese history.]

[Footnote 4: The imperial pronoun "Tchin," *me*, is with very good taste supplied by *I* in these impassioned passages.]

ACT THIRD

Enter Envoy, escorting the Princess, with a band of music.

PRINCESS. Thus was I, in spite of the treachery of Maouyenshow, who disfigured my portrait, seen and exalted by his Majesty; but the traitor presented a truer likeness to the Tartar king, who comes at the head of an army to demand me, with a threat of seizing the country. There is no remedy—I must be yielded up to propitiate the invaders! How shall I bear the rigors—the winds and frosts of that foreign land! It has been said of old, that "surpassing beauty is often coupled with an unhappy fate." Let me grieve, then, without entertaining fruitless resentment at the effects of my own attractions.

Enter Emperor, attended by his several officers.

EMPEROR. This day we take leave of the princess at Pahling bridge! [*To his ministers.*] Can ye not devise a way to send out these foreign troops, without yielding up the princess for the sake of peace? [*Descends from his horse and seems to grieve with Chaoukeun.*] Let our attendants delay awhile, till we have conferred the parting cup.

ENVOY. Lady, let us urge you to proceed on your way—the sky darkens, and night is coming on.

PRINCESS. Alas! when shall I again behold your Majesty? I will take off my robes of distinction and leave them behind me. To-day in the palace of Han—to-morrow I shall be espoused to a stranger. I cease to wear these splendid vestments—they shall no longer adorn my beauty in the eyes of men.

ENVOY. Again let us urge you, princess, to depart; we have delayed but too long already!

EMPEROR. 'Tis done!—Princess, when you are gone, let your thoughts forbear to dwell with sorrow and resentment upon us! [*They part.*] And am I the great Monarch of the line of Han?

PRESIDENT. Let your Majesty cease to dwell with such grief upon this subject!

EMPEROR. She is gone! In vain have we maintained those armed heroes on the frontier. [1] Mention but swords and spears, and they tremble at their hearts like a young deer. The princess has this day performed what belonged to themselves: and yet they affect the semblance of men!

PRESIDENT. Your Majesty is entreated to return to the palace: dwell not so bitterly, Sir, on her memory:—allow her to depart!

EMPEROR. Did I not think of her, I had a heart of iron—a heart of iron! The tears of my grief stream in thousand channels—this evening shall her likeness be suspended in the palace, where I will sacrifice to it—and tapers with their silver lights shall illuminate her chamber.

PRESIDENT. Let your Majesty return to the palace—the princess is already far distant! [*Exeunt.*

The Tartar Camp. Enter K'han at the head of his tribes, leading in the Princess.

K'HAN. The Emperor of Han having now, in observance of old treaties, yielded up to me the Lady Chaoukeun in marriage, I take her as my rightful queen. The two nations shall enjoy the benefits of peace. [*To his generals*] Leaders, transmit my commands to the army to strike our encampment, and proceed to the north. [*They march.*

The river Amoor. [2] Tartar army on its march.

PRINCESS. What place is this?

ENVOY. It is the River of the Black Dragon, the frontier of the Tartar territories and those of China. This southern shore is the Emperor's; on the northern side commences our Tartar dominion.

PRINCESS [*to the K'han*]. Great King, I take a cup of wine, and pour a libation towards the South—my last farewell to the Emperor—[*pours the libation*] of Han, this life is finished. I await thee in the next!

[*Throws herself into the river. The K'han, in great consternation, endeavors to save her, but in vain.*

K'HAN. Alas! alas!—so determined was her purpose against this foreign alliance—she has thrown herself into the stream, and perished! Tis done, and remediless! Let her sepulchre be on this river's bank, and be it called "the verdant tomb," [3] She is no more; and vain has been our enmity with the dynasty of Han! The traitor Maouyenshow was the author of all this misery. [*To an officer*] Take Maouyenshow and let him be delivered over to the Emperor for punishment. I will return to our former friendship with the dynasty of Han. We will renew and long preserve the sentiments of relationship. The traitor disfigured the portrait to injure Chaoukeun—then deserted his sovereign, and stole over to me, whom he prevailed on to demand the lady in marriage. How little did I think that she would thus precipitate herself into the stream, and perish!—In vain did my spirit melt at the sight of her! But if I detained this profligate and traitorous rebel, he would certainly prove to us a root of misfortune: it is better to deliver him for his reward to the Emperor of Han, with whom I will renew, and long retain, our old feelings of friendship and amity. *[Exeunt.*

[Footnote 1: It may be observed that the great wall is never once expressly mentioned through this drama. The expression used is Peensih, the border, or frontier. The wall had existed two hundred years at this time, but the real frontier was beyond it.]

[Footnote 2: Or Saghalien, which falls into the sea of Ochotsk.]

[Footnote 3: Said to exist now and to be green all the year.]

ACT FOURTH

Enter Emperor, with an attendant.

EMPEROR. Since the princess was yielded to the Tartars, we have not held an audience. The lonely silence of night but increases our melancholy! We take the picture of that fair one and suspend it here, as some small solace to our griefs, [*To the attendant*] Keeper of the yellow gate, behold, the incense in yonder vase is burnt out: hasten then to add some more. Though we cannot see her, we may at least retain this shadow; and, while life remains, betoken our regard. But oppressed and weary, we would fain take a little repose.

[*Lies down to sleep. The Princess appears before him in a vision.*] [1]

PRINCESS. Delivered over as a captive to appease the barbarians, they would have conveyed me to their Northern country: but I took an occasion to elude them and have escaped back. Is not this the Emperor, my sovereign? Sir, behold me again restored.

[*A Tartar soldier appears in the vision.*]

SOLDIER. While I chanced to sleep, the lady, our captive, has made her escape, and returned home. In eager pursuit of her, I have reached the imperial palace.—Is not this she?

[*Carries her off. The Emperor starts from his sleep.*]

EMPEROR. We just saw the Princess returned—but alas, how quickly has she vanished! In bright day she answered not to our call—but when morning dawned on our troubled sleep, a vision presented her in this spot. [*Hears the wild fowl's [2] cry*] Hark, the passing fowl screamed twice or thrice!—Can it know there is no one so desolate as I? [*Cries repeated*] Perhaps worn out and weak, hungry and emaciated, they bewail at once the broad nets of the South and the tough bows of the North. [*Cries repeated*] The screams of those water-birds but increase our melancholy.

ATTENDANT. Let your Majesty cease this sorrow, and have some regard to your sacred [3] person.

EMPEROR. My sorrows are beyond control. Cease to upbraid this excess of feeling, since ye are all subject to the same. Yon doleful cry is not the note of the swallow on the carved rafters, nor the song of the variegated bird upon the blossoming tree. The princess has abandoned her home! Know ye in what place she grieves, listening like me to the screams of the wild bird?

Enter President.

PRESIDENT. This day after the close of the morning council, a foreign envoy appeared, bringing with him the fettered traitor Maouyenshow. He announces that the renegade, by deserting his allegiance, led to the breach of truce, and occasioned all these calamities. The princess is no more! and the K'han wishes for peace and friendship between the two nations. The envoy attends, with reverence, your imperial decision.

EMPEROR. Then strike off the traitor's head, and be it presented as an offering to the shade of the princess! Let a fit banquet be got ready for the envoy, preparatory to his return. *[Recites these verses.*

At the fall of the leaf, when the wild-fowl's cry was heard
    in the recesses of the palace.
Sad dreams returned to our lonely pillow; we thought of
    her through the night:
Her verdant tomb remains—but where shall we seek her

self?
The perfidious painter's head shall atone for the beauty
which he wronged.

[Footnote 1: There is nothing in this more extravagant than the similar vision in the tragedy of Richard III.]

[Footnote 2: Yengo, a species of wild goose, is the emblem in China of intersexual attachment and fidelity, being said never to pair again after the loss of its mate. An image of it is worshipped by newly married couples.]

[Footnote 3: Literally, "dragon person." The emperor's throne is often called the "dragon seat."]

Made in the USA
Monee, IL
13 September 2026

62976981R00154